FEAR DIFFERENTIAL

Gene Cardema

CONTENTS

Dedication

This novel is written in honor of the nurses who sacrificed and lost their lives in the service during the covid pandemic. This book is dedicated to all the nurses I worked with who have poured their energies to the care of the countless patients who have come to seek treatment for cancer. Their devotion to a higher standard of patient care is commendable and worthy of respect.

ACKNOWLEDGEMENTS

Acknowledgement

I am grateful to the Directing Intelligence who guided me to write this novel starting from the outline from which the storyline flowed from. This book is not written by AI or influenced by it in any means or manner. It is an organic composition stemming from years of experience working as a nurse.

I give thanks to the medical institution that gave me the opportunity to grow in my profession and kept me gainfully employed through unstable times. My heartfelt thanks to Northeastern University and the professors – Dr. Jane Aroian, Dr. Lynn Babbington - who have shown me the way through the gates of higher learning.

No disrespect to judge Judy for mentioning her name. I extend my apologies for any misconception.

And lastly, I acknowledge the wealth of information from online sources from which I gathered all the selected data cited in this book.

Print information available on the last page.
ISBN: 979-8-7652-6582-6 (sc)
ISBN: 979-8-7652-6581-9 (e)
Library of Congress Control Number: 202591910

Chapter One

BLOOD, SWEAT, AND FEARS

7:00 am. The wall clock above her patient's bed chimed. My shift is done, Maria told herself gladly as she hurried to hang her last IV antibiotics on her patient in room 301. It's late, was due for 6 am but she was swarmed with other tasks the 12-hour shift went fast. She had no time for it except now, not even time for bathroom break. Her bladder was full, her stomach's empty, but she has to prioritize her patient's needs before her own. Her other patient has a hematocrit of 24. She was ordered a bag of blood but the lady at the blood bank yelled at her gruffly, "it's not ready yet," When she called 3x. The next nurse would just have to deal with it. Maria didn't care how her replacement would fuss and fume but at this point she didn't give a hoot. She was just relieved her work was over. Her shift may be over however, unbeknownst to her the nightmare was just about to begin.

She stepped out of the patient's room in 301 and found the hallway, the nurse's station, even the med room empty. Maria sensed a 'disturbance in the field'. What happened to the staff? Where did all the nurses go? She wondered. It's eerily quiet except for a hissing sound coming from the other side of the unit where the last rooms 310, 309, 308 are located. She followed the source of the god-awful sound and was shocked to find the 3 patients out of their rooms, two were sprawled on the floor unconsciously lying in their own piss and vomit. The third patient was slouched, leaning on the beige wall now red from her own blood. Her whole body in major convulsion shaking and spewing out more blood from her blocked nostrils creating a hissing noise. Maria hopscotched in between limbs careful not to step on the green gooey fluid that came out of the patient's mouth.

How did these patients come out of the isolation rooms? She stooped down to feel their pulses. One was dead, the other dying with faint pulse and barely breathing. The third patient was still alive drowning in his own secretions. She heard a door opening and from room 306 came out another covid casualty with her IV lines entangled around her, cut off from the IV bag leaking black fluid all over the floor as she zombied out of her room.

Where did the staff go? She yelled on top of her lungs.

"Help!! Anybody in here?", but she found herself alone except for the dead, the dying and the walking dead. There's nobody in the unit to help her. This can't be happening she told herself as fear pumped up in her veins with wild abandon.

Maria was no stranger to fear. In her 25 years of her nursing career, she knew of it as a raging monster that wreaked havoc in her insides; sometimes a nauseated feeling that cannot be denied; oftentimes just cold sweats trickling down her back; at times her heart galloping like an untamed horse trying to bust out of her chest. In her years of working at the BMT/ICU unit for 20 years she learned to tame it and gave it a different spin. She tells herself, what is fear but a swarm of hungry butterflies fluttering in her insides, a not-so-gentle flutter in her gut running up and down her spine. This time, fear came out as angry bats flocking all over her as the door in room 305 opened and another patient came out naked, grotesquely disfigured covered in cuts and weeping warts heading to where she was.

Now she's in pure panic. Terrified, she bolted up and run towards the North exit by room 301 but outside the double doors there were 11 half-dead patients milling around just waiting for someone to open it. She turned and bee-lined to the other exit on the south side of the unit and as she cut through the darkened storage room, she felt a cold wet hand grabbed her ankle. She tripped on someone lying in between the storage racks. He mumbled weakly,

"Help."

She could barely see his face but she recognized the voice as her other patient in room 304.

"Vincent, how did you get in here?"

She lost her balance and now she's down on the floor, too, beside him. Terror filled her whole being as he was about to climb over her, his bodily fluids seeping into her scrubs. She closed her eyes tightly and yelled.

"God get me out of here!!!"

Overwhelmed with so much fear, she heard a loud alarm. She opened her eyes and realized she's lying in her own bed drenched in her own sweat. She started crying, sobbing her eyes out. Tears of relief and sweat swamped her pillow. Thank God it was just a nightmare. The alarm was from the clock at her bedside table set for 5:00 pm. She must have pushed the snooze button to sleep a little bit more. She was so exhausted coming home from her 1st 12-hour shift last night that she slept through the day. The nightmare woke her up. She was languishing on the disturbing images when she heard a voice.

"Maria, wake up. I'll meet you on the other side of fear."

Where did that come from, she wondered. And what did it mean?

It's now 6:20 pm, for sure she would be late for the 7 pm shift. She hurried to get ready for another long shift at the coal mine as she preferred to name the hospital. To her it is the dark underbelly of health care.

Maria lived in the outskirts of Boston in a suburb named after the valley of the roses few miles south of the main hub. It's still part of the city but without the traffic and congestion in the jumbled disorganized streets of Beantown, a best forgotten moniker for Boston attributed to several tales. One was from the early settlers – the Puritans, mainly subsisting on beans slow-baked in molasses. Another was from the transiting sailors and merchant marines enjoying the quick cheap meal of beans. A third tale was from the city dwellers having bad flatulence inhaling the dirty water from the once filthiest harbor in the U.S. Now the harbor had been cleaned up and she loved the seaport side, dirty or not. She's glad she came to Beantown and found the right place to work at – the esteemed research institution of St. Johnswart with 800 beds split up in different services and medical specialties.

Her commute to the hospital was the best part of her shift as she drove by the Arnold arboretum- a 365-acre wooded oasis in the midst of urban setting. From the energy of the trees, she filled herself with the stamina to endure the long shifts at the covid unit. Arborway, the road that runs along the north end of the arboretum, takes her to a rotary before it merges with Jamaicaway. Jamaicaway is a slithering street that bends and curves under the canopy of trees lining the eastern part of Jamaica Pond – a glacial 'kettle lake' that empties into the Charles River. It's a watering hole for ducks and men that fish the shallow reservoir.

The ancient mighty oaks arising from the undulating grounds in the south side of the pond are living testament of nature's resilience to the harsh New England Winters and where she draws her strength from to do her work. In Autumn, the red and gold foliage around the pond reflected in the water elevates the place into an ethereal realm. Right now, in the middle of January, the trees are frozen; life suspended to rest for the season.

The 25-minute drive to the hospital was less harried on her side of the road while on the other side of the yellow lane, cars piled up in the narrow curving road of Jamaica Way. People were coming home from their day job, while she's on her way to her graveyard shift. She wondered why it's called graveyard shift? Maybe because the hospital is a holding yard for people before they head on to their graves. Most escape the holding cell, summoned by fate to live a little bit longer or maybe just lucky to be home with family. But some unfortunate ones succumbed to unscheduled death for relatives to weep through an unexpected funeral.

"Why are you so grim?" she chided herself and banged her head lightly on the steering wheel, her car stopped on the red light waiting for it to change. She can wait here forever if it's up to her. She reached her saturation point in her nursing career where she's ready to just quit and walk away. The car behind her honked before the light turned green.

"Fuck off!", she blasted her horn back.

Maria didn't really want to go to work but at thirty minutes before the shift, it's too late to call in sick. She was still reeling from the nightmare as she drove on to the hospital. She hoped it's not a dream rehearsal for the real nightmare that oftentimes unfold during a 12-hour shift at the Covid mine. She hurried on towards Riverway, a meandering drive that flanks the west and top of the Longwood Medical and Academic area.

The Longwood area is home to colleges and universities, one of which is the prestigious Harvard Medical School. There's a conglomeration of renowned medical institutions that are mostly the training ground for Harvard medical students. The collection of reputable hospitals jampacked in a small plotted piece of real estate includes Children's Hospital, consistently the top pediatric hospital in the nation. Five others are clustered in the medical mecca. Not included in the Longwood area farther northeast close to the Charles River is Massachusetts General Hospital. Founded in 1811, it is the 3rd oldest general hospital in the United States. It is where the first anesthesia was used and where anesthesiology was born.

From Riverway Maria veered right on to Brookline Avenue and turned into the parking garage. She entered the rear entrance of the building hoping the line to get into the elevator would not be as long. The 'gatekeeper' at the foyer handing out synthetic masks to every one entering, asked her gruffly.

"Your Id, ma'am?"

Maria rummaged inside her work bag as he barked at her impatiently.

"Hurry, you're holding the line", and stick a digital thermometer in her forehead. "98.1, you're good to go".

"Oh, great, I'm still alive", she mumbled with sarcasm.

She headed to follow the yellow round markers six feet apart, laid out in fine Italian marble before it stops right in front of the elevator. The wall clock above it says 10 minutes past 7 pm. She's late but glad she missed the elevator rush hour. There were 4 young nurses in blue scrubs before her with their chin to their chest, I-phone in hand, face booking to while away the wait. The elevator opened up and 6 haggardly looking nurses came out, their scrubs soiled and their faces wearing the butts they must have cleaned in their own shifts that just ended.

She got off the elevator on the 3rd floor, turned right on the hallway towards the west wing of the building. The double door electronic entrance to the unit has a big orange hexagonal sign that says, 'STOP'. Underneath spells 'SPU- Special Pathogens Unit'. The sign looked foreboding enough that if you have any sense at all you'd walk away. There's nothing special about it, only a dark vault – a mausoleum that housed the living dead. Maria wanted to paste a banner below it that says. 'Covid Unit- Enter at your own risk.' She took a deep breath and exclaimed to herself.

"Here we go. Let the stress begin!" She pushed the metal button on the right side of the door to open up to the south side of the unit where room 301 was situated. She hoped she'll have the same patient that was there last night but the room was empty.

"Hey Lauren, what happened to my patient in 301?" she asked the day charge nurse giving report to Mindy, the incoming charge nurse. Both sitting in front of room 302.

"She died." She said with a stone-cold face.

"What? When? She was fine for me last night. What happened? She's only 24!" Maria barraged her with questions but she brushed her off.

"You are late!" she scolded her. "Go find Cecil, she's waiting for you. You have 2 patients for now till you get an admission in 301."

Cecil was standing impatiently by the nurse's station with her jacket on, her bag on her right shoulder, ready to leave. She handed Maria a tiny piece of paper.

"Here's a list of what else is left to do for your patients. I didn't have time for it." Maria asked flabbergasted, still processing the fact that her patient in 301 is gone, "What's this? where's the rest of the report?" Cecil retorted as she walked away, "Go dig EPIC, I gotta go. I have to pick up my son from day care. My husband can't do it. Good luck with your shift."

EPIC is the branded EMR (electronic medical record) recently acquired by the hospital for efficient tracking of medical information. It contains everything you want to know about a patient – their personal, medical, physical history. It's a convenient tool for Billings department to charge patients for their entire hospital stay; a digital akashic record with so many layers and domain that you need more than half a brain to navigate it. The young nurses take to it like ducks to water. They're most savvy at navigating the medical hyperspace while the older generation of nurses dread it to the point of retirement. Another strategy to save on labor cost; get rid of nurses on higher pay scale.

She logged into the computer and looked at the med list, the day's lab results and what tasks need to be done during her shift. Patient in 303 – Lisa Brooks- has a K of 3.1, her Mg is 1.5 and needed to be replaced. Mrs. Donnovan in 304 needs platelets and a bag of red cell.

"What did Cecil do all day?" Maria complained to the charge nurse.

"She just coded her patient in 301 for 3 hours," Mindy replied back.

After reading the patient's profile, Maria proceeded to the med room adjacent to the nurse's station to gather all the meds needed for her 2 patients when Mindy, yelled.

"Maria, you have an admission in 301. ER nurse is on line 1 for report."

"Cripes, the room is still warm from the previous patient, her ghost is still there hanging around. Let it cool off." She muttered to herself. She kept her sarcasm instead and asked Mindy.

"Can you give it to another nurse. I haven't done assessment on my patients yet."

"I'll take report for you but you have to take this patient." she replied. "Carol and Camille already have their 3 patients."

The night staff consists of two aids, three nurses with 3 patients each, and the charge nurse with one patient to help around and support the three nurses. When the pandemic first started, patient nurse ratio was 1:1, but as the staff got more proficient with the isolation protocol, it became 2:1. Now, each nurse has three patients as the novelty of it all wore off.

"How does it sound on paper"? Maria asked.

"Not too bad." She replied. "44, Spanish speaking lady, had 102.5 fever at home with difficulty breathing. The husband brought her to the emergency room. How's your Spanish?" she asked.

"Me? Maria maybe my name but no habla Espanol. Un pokito maybe. I hope she doesn't come before I assess my two patients."

Maria gathered the paraphernalia needed to enter the isolation rooms-- goggles, plastic shield, N-95 face mask, puke buckets to place them all on top of the side table right outside the patient's room. It has 3 drawers where the yellow disposable gowns are stored. She can garb up now by herself without help from an aid, but when the pandemic first started, it took two people to follow the protocol to enter a Covid isolation room. Once you're in, if you forget something, you just can't go out again to fetch anything without having to go through the process all over again. You press the help button and someone will slide it through a box built into the wall with an opening on both the outside and the inside. The patient rooms are equipped with medical supplies - alcohol wipes, syringes, thermometers but if the previous shift used it all up without restocking, you'll be fuming and cussing behind the suffocating mask.

She entered room 303 armored like a cop facing a street protester. The string of her mask snapped and riding up to her eye google behind the plastic shield,

"Shit, not a good start to my shift," she mumbled to herself, as she rummaged through the supply cart looking for a stethoscope.

"Hi Maria, I'm glad to see you again. Are you my nurse for tonight?" asked Lisa in between coughing fits.

"Hello Lisa, yes. I am. I see you need some cough medicine. Can you push your call button?"

"How can I help you?", the secretary at the desk answered the call.

"Hey Patty, can you ask another nurse to grab some cough medicine and Albuterol from the Omnicell? It's for Ms. Brooks and get me another N-95, will you?"

She listened to her chest and upper back and her lungs sounded like a washing machine. She's surprised her finger oximeter was reading 92%. Her heart was compensating to work harder as evidenced by her pulse rate fluctuating from 120-130 per minute showing on the cardiac monitor. For her own sanity she'd like her pulse below 110 so she doesn't have to hear the alarms going off every time the parameters are breached over 120. She piggy-backed the Magnesium in her main IV line after she gave her the nebulizer treatment.

"Lisa, call when the nebulizer is done. I will be back to hang your Potassium. I just have to see my other patient."

As she was about to enter her 2nd patient in 304, her admission was wheeled in. "Holy crap, I guess Mrs. Donnovan will just have to wonder who her night nurse might be."

The two ER nurses calmly deposited the new patient, Mrs. Lina Alvarez to her room in 301. They were fully garbed up in Hazmat suits as they transported the patient from the ED, radiating an aura of the stoic warriors fighting the unseen enemy. They masterfully hauled her from the stretcher to the bed, switched the oxygen from the portable cylinder to the wall unit and hooked her to the cardiac monitor while Maria suited up to follow them, her nerves starting to fray before entering the room.

"She's only on 4 liters of Oxygen for now but you might need to call the respiratory guy for a Hi-flow set up." The older ER nurse told Maria.

She has seen many Covid patients in the ER and from experience, she knew patient can go from bad to worse in a flash.

"Right now, I'm not thinking about Hi-flow set up, just mentally brushing up on few Spanish words I know."

The patient looked so anxious and breathing hard. Maria thought to herself, she definitely needs an order for Lorazepam IV. One for her and one for me.

"Ola, mi llamo Maria. No habla Espanol but un pokito, si senora?"

She smiled faintly and relaxed a bit, as she settled back on her bed cranked up 45 degrees. Mindy came through the intercom.

"I paged the admitting resident. He's on his way to see her."

She was doing the initial assessment from head to toe when he came in the room. Maria entered her admission data into the Epic system quickly and tried to do as much computer work before the resident takes complete control of the machine for his own admitting info.

"Ola, I'm Dr. Chavez, I and Maria will be taking care of you tonight."

He must have looked at the assignment board and learned who's taking care of who. From all the protective gear he's wearing-- yellow gown, googles, mask, face shield and green OR cap, she couldn't tell what ethnic background he might be. Maria thought to herself.

'Chavez? What are the chances that he speaks Spanish more than I do? I don't' see him using a google translator, so I hoped he does speak it more fluent than my broken Spanglish.'

Thank heavens he does!

"Sorry to interrupt, do you want another bag of Lactated Ringers on her?" Maria asked the doctor pointing to the current IV bag running that's almost empty.

"Her blood pressure is better now." She indicated to the resident.

The recent BP reading on the monitor shows 100/60. It was below 90 systolic when she was at the ED.

"No. She has a cardiac history. Just run maintenance fluids after this bag, Normal saline at 50cc an hour", he said finishing his physical assessment.

"Can I ask a favor?" Maria asked him. "I know it's beneath your scope of practice but before you go out, can you show her how the bed control works and tell her that I'll be watching her through that window," pointing to the square glass aperture on the right side of the door. It has blinds that can be controlled from a small alcove built into the wall outside each room that houses the monitor and computer above the counter where nurses sit to give report.

"Gladly, Maria." He said, "page me if you need anything."

After wrapping up her admission, Maria went to see her 3rd patient.

"Hello Mrs. Donovan, sorry it took me awhile to get in here."

No response. Her vital signs showing on the monitor looked fine, she must be in deep sleep, she thought. She's not connected to anything except the monitor wires and her IV line hanging on the pole. She pulled the covers to access her central line to connect her to the IV tubing.

She gasped, "Holy Shit." The patient was lying unconscious on a pool of blood coming from her double lumen Hickman. She pushed the call light hurriedly.

"Can I help you?" Mindy answered the call from the desk.

"Come quick, help me apply pressure dressing on her, she's bleeding from her Hickman. Ask someone to get her bag of blood and platelets! Pronto." Maria nervously yelled, as she flattened her palms on her chest to stop the blood gushing from underneath the dressing of the central line.

Mrs. Donovan, at 52, was recently diagnosed with AML (acute myelogenous leukemia) and was scheduled for induction chemotherapy but she turned positive for

Covid. She was transferred from the Heme/Onc. unit with a freshly minted central line. Her platelets and hematocrit are low, needing transfusions almost every other day. But today because of the code she wasn't transfused promptly.

Having her as a patient reminded her of her days working in the bone marrow transplant unit where most of the patients were diagnosed with AML (acute myelogenous leukemia) and ALL (acute lymphocytic leukemia). AML is a type of blood cancer where the bone marrow produces immature white blood cells called blasts proliferating in the blood stream. The circulating blasts crowd the red cells, white blood cells and platelets rendering them dysfunctional. Thus, the body becomes susceptible to infection, bleeding and fatigue. It's caused by chemicals like benzene, pesticides, cleaning products, paint strippers as well as exposure to radiation and chemotherapy such as Cytoxan, Melphalan, Doxorubicin and Mitoxantrone. Treatment starts with Induction chemotherapy to kill the leukemic cells followed by consolidation; more chemo to eradicate the residual cancer cells to achieve remission. Then a stem cell or bone marrow transplant is undertaken by those who choose to do it as recommended by the oncologists. Taking care of her triggered memories of her working as a transplant nurse.

"Oh, hi girls." Mrs. Donnovan opened her eyes as Mindy and Maria were finishing to change her bed sheets. "When did you get here? I must have slept so soundly. I was dreaming I was in Aruba lying on a warm sand".

Maria wanted to tell her, "The warmth you felt was from your blood you're soaked in."

Instead, she said,

"Welcome back Eilleen, Aruba is much better than here. Boston is frozen in the middle of January. I'm sure you wished you were still there when you woke up."

When the blood products arrived, she practically pushed the 150cc bag of platelets through her central line and ran the red blood cells faster than policy dictates. She tolerated it fine and actually needed a second bag of red cell after all the blood she lost.

Maria hasn't eaten anything before she came to work as she slept through the whole day. She was in the backroom behind the nurse's station halfway through an old sandwich left over from the previous shift when the aid popped in.

"Your patient in 303 is calling."

"Can you ask one of the nurses to go in? I just want to finish this sandwich," Maria told the aid.

"They're all in their patient's rooms." She said, "Besides she specifically asked for you", she added.

Lisa was a young, 23 years old student studying to be a nurse at Boston university. She had her last night, too, so she got attached to her. She didn't want anybody to answer her call except for Maria. She walked into her room and saw soiled Kleenex strewn all over the floor. Every time she coughed and spit out phlegm on a tissue, she threw them on the floor. The room was littered with covid bombs, a perfect poster ad for a freaking SPP, 'special pathogen paradise'. Her cough and wheezing were better after the nebulizer but now has a temperature of 101.5 F.

"I feel cold", she said starting to shake raising her heart rate even higher—130-140/minute, the alarms on her heart monitor ringing incessantly. Maria called for a warm blanket, but warm blankets from the machine don't stay warm for long. She cranked up the thermostat in the room and now she herself was dying inside the yellow gown, suffocating behind the mask and face shield, feeling faint as sweats from her armpits trickled down her sides. Her body heat was trapped in the synthetic yellow gown wrapped tightly around her. With the thermostat up in the 80's, she was cramped in the living inferno she was in.

"Oh God," she prayed. "Don't let me pass out in here." She remembered the prayer her mother taught her that always works when she finds herself in a bind. "I can do all things through Christ which gives me strength and power. I can do all things through Christ which gives me strength and power."

Mindy's voice came through the intercom, "Maria, what can I do for you?", she asked.

"Page the doctor for a Demerol order, she's shaking bad even with 5 blankets on her." She replied.

Demerol is not only a potent pain medicine but also stops the rigors effectively. After a moment that felt like eternity, trying to console the shivering little Lisa, scared out of her wits, Mindy slid the 25 mgs. Demerol bristoject through the box.

"How much did he order?" she asked.

"A whole 6.25 mg of it," Mindy replied with sarcasm.

"What? That's just piss in the wind," Maria said exasperated. Lisa was shaking badly now, her teeth chattering, her fragile bones rattling as she's shaking wildly under the cover.

"I'm so scared, can you make it stop?" Lisa whimpered.

Maria hunched over her like a mother hen protecting her young.

"It will be over soon Lisa, just breathe deeply." Finally, Lisa stopped shaking after she pushed the Demerol.,

"That was fast. The 6.25 mg worked?" Mindy asked watching through the glass panel.

"Not really. My finger just slipped, ooppps." Maria replied.

Mindy smiled knowingly in approval.

The resident came in, ordered triple IV antibiotics after 2 sets of blood cultures. Maria was hesitating on telling him but she did it anyway.

"Hey doc, the 6.25 mg did not work. She was shaking so bad I had to give the whole bristoject. Can you order the 25mg.?"

"Sure. You got it."

She was relieved, as she thought he would be mad.

'Judge Judy won't be going after me,' she told herself. 'At least, what I did is now legal'.

She acknowledged to herself, 'Sometimes you got lucky when you work with doctors with a little less ego and more respect for the nurses working on the trenches of the covid battle field.'

Lisa was snoring after the Demerol. Maria got the blood cultures from her Hickman line before she left the room. Every time she drew blood from a central line there's always that apprehension that she needed to overcome. She carefully transferred the blood into the culture bottles, labeled them, sent them off to the lab via the pneumatic tube then proceeded back to her remaining sandwich and hoped she could have a quiet break. Carol and Camille joined her coming back from the cafeteria.

"Hey, did you hear if the contract settled. The MNA (Massachusetts Nurses Association) proposed a 2% raise". Camille started.

"No," Carol replied. "The hospital administration's refusing to budge. We've been working for two years now, still under the old contract. The MNA wants to raise the night shift differential to $1.75 an hour and the charge differential up to 2 dollars."

Aside from the base rate, nurses are paid additional shift differential for working the evening, night and weekends shifts. The charge nurses are compensated more for the responsibility of managing the unit and the staff.

"By the way," Camille interjected, "They posted a new permanent charge position, why don't you apply Maria?"

"Thanks, but no thanks. Two dollars an hour is not even worth the headache of being in charge of the chaos around here. Headache differential, I call it. You can't tag a dollar amount for the crap you have to deal with. Ask Mindy, she's been doing charge most of the time, might as well make it official."

Maria was on her last bite of her sandwich when the alarm from the central monitor broke their break time.

"Oh, now what?" Maria muttered chomping off the last remaining piece of the bread as she looked at the central monitor in the nurse's station. Her new patient in 301 has a heart rate of 140/minute, her oxygen saturation fluctuated between 88-89% on 4 Liters of Oxygen. She hurried into her room to check maybe the finger oximeter was just misaligned in her index finger. She's coughing hard and breathing harder now as she gets more anxious. Maria dialed up her oxygen to 6 liters. She yelled for Mindy through the intercom.

"Can you page the doctor? She needs breathing treatment and a shot of Ativan".

Dr. Chavez came in, listen to her lungs, shook his head as he hung his stethoscope out of habit around his neck.

"She's got fluids in her lungs now, she sounded clear when she first came in", he said. "Give her nebulizer every 4 hours and Lasix to diurese her. Keep her saturation above 90 %."

"Can I place a foley catheter on her?" Maria asked. "What about some Ativan? She's very anxious, her anxiety exacerbates her breathing and her heart rate".

"Give her 0.25 mg. now. We don't want to sedate her too much, and it's a no on the foley", he said as he walked towards the door.

"She'll be groggy from the Ativan to walk to the bathroom and with the Lasix, she'll be peeing up a storm." Maria argued. "She's very weak to begin with." Despite her best effort, Maria lost her case on the foley catheter.

"Get her a bedside commode then. No catheter for now", he said emphatically.

Lasix is a diuretic named appropriately as its effects last for six hours. Maria would be bailing out the Hoover dam with thousands of covid bugs swimming around. And for the next six hours, she and Lina would be tripping to the bathroom frequently after all the fluids she had been pumped up at the ED.

"Fine", Maria grumbled "Oh, by the way, don't walk away with the stethoscope unless you want to spread Covid all over the hospital." Maria barked at him, miffed because he refused to order a foley catheter.

With six liters of oxygen via nasal prong her saturation reading went up to 92%. Her heart rate is down to 110 after the shot of Ativan.

'No, I did not let my fingers slip on the bristoject this time.' Maria was thinking out loud as if addressing judge Judy. The small dose is enough to relax her but she needs to be awake enough to breathe. Too much narcotic depresses the respiratory drive.

Maria was about to make rounds for the 12 midnight meds when the call light from room 301 came on.

"El bano." She said weakly through the intercom.

Then all hell broke loose. The alarms from her monitor were ringing mercilessly amplified by the bed alarm. Maria knew when the diuretic starts to take effect she'll be getting on her own to the bathroom, but she's too weak to get up by herself so she activated the bed alarm. She was too late. By the time she was done gowning up, before she can get inside the room, Lina already untangled herself from the wires and halfway to the bathroom she fell down alongside the IV pole with two pumps tied in it, missing her by this much; the T-shape metal pole six inches away from her head. A mini-deluge of covid-infested piss flooded half of the room. Mindy came in to help her shuffled Lina back to bed. Lina was huffing and puffing, and with the supply of oxygen cut off for the brief time she was out of bed, her finger oximeter was reading 86%. Maria turned the Oxygen meter up to 8 Liters but her saturation just went up to 89%. The ER nurse was right. She would eventually need a Hi-flow set up to deliver more oxygen in her lungs.

The resident came in, checked the patient and cleared her for possible injuries. There's a worried line on his forehead as he wrote several orders; change of Oxygen from nasal prong to Hi-flow, more Lasix to dry out Lina's lungs and the coveted foley catheter!

Maria wanted to say, "I told you so".

The unit settled down after 1 am. With all the 10 patients tucked in, the nurses went back to eating what remains of their supper.

"Maria, are you caught up?" Mindy asked. "What can I help you with?"

"I just need to catch up on documentation and do the stupid incident report. Thank God Lina wasn't hurt during the fall."

Of all the things Maria hated the most, it's doing an incident report. It's not the paper work itself but the implication behind it. It makes her feel incompetent and negligent of her duties. She can deal with different emergency codes-- green, blue, brown, but having a patient fall on her shift was something she abhorred. Code green is when a patient's blood pressure drops to dangerous level with a sustained tachycardia not resolved right away. Code blue is more serious with a respiratory component and an impending threat of death. Code brown is the 'clean-up in aisle 7' kind of emergency, not serious at all but it's the second thing she hated.

She remembered many moons ago working on the BMT unit, she had a confused patient high risk for fall. A bedside commode was placed in her room to keep her from trailing brown liquid diarrhea from bed to bathroom but she's refusing to use it. The sitter went on break so Maria sat right outside the curtain that provided privacy to the patient inside a glass walled room. Maria heard the bed creaked and the sound of the commode being pushed away, the aluminum legs screeching against the floor. She rushed into the room, saw the patient getting out of bed heading for the bathroom. Maria pointed her index finger at her like cocking a gun and said to her menacingly,

"Freeze."

The patient froze, with her right foot in front of the other as she was about to walk to the bathroom. She was confused and catatonic now, not moving at all. Brown liquid flowed out of her rear end like a cascading waterfall streaming down the sides and back of her legs down to the floor in copious amount. When she moved, she slipped and sprawled on the slimy floor. Maria had to call for a code brown; clean up in room 11.

Her reverie was broken by the alarm from room 301. The monitor is showing 85% oxygen saturation and a heart rate of 150-160. Mindy paged the resident and the respiratory therapist stat as Maria rushed into room 301. Lina was breathing so hard on 50% Hi-flow. She's very anxious, rambling in Spanish Maria couldn't understand.

"Calmante Lina, breathe, respirar por favor."

Maria's grappling for Spanish words to calm her down and felt helpless, not being able to communicate. She held her hand reassuringly as she herself was deep breathing to prompt Lina, showing her how to do it, to no avail. Lina was gasping for air, her lips turning blue as her oxygen level dropped below the low normal of 90%, down to 82-80-78%. Her heart rate went the opposite direction, up to 170-180/minute. The alarms were nerve-wracking but Maria's own deep breathing calmed herself down as fear started to creep up her spine.

"Shit, shit, shit. She's gonna code", says her anxious, nervous alter ego, exacerbated by the blaring alarms.

"No, she's not," says a small voice in her head. "Stay calm. You have the power to control the situation. You got this."

The respiratory therapist came before the resident, dialed up her Oxygen to 80% and increased the pressure. Lina started to slow down her breathing as her saturation went up to 88% and color came back to her lips. She needed that pressurized high concentrated oxygen to flood her lungs and her bloodstream. Her heart rate though was up to 200/minute with irregular heartbeat, the monitor in constantly alarming tachycardia. Maria yelled at Mindy standing by outside 301.

"Where is Dr. Chavez? What is taking him so long? Shall we call a code?"

"He's here now, just ordered Metoprolol IV. I'll give it to you as soon as it's ordered", Mindy replied back and asked "What's her pressure?"

Maria cycled the automatic BP on the cardiac monitor every 10 minutes.

"It's 88/58 right now. The Metoprolol will drop down her blood pressure even lower."

"I just ordered 2.5 mg. to slow down her heart rate", said the doctor as he came into the room. "If her BP goes down, we'll just give her more fluids."

"Hopefully not", Maria quipped back. "I just drained her lungs. I hate to pump more fluids on her. I don't understand, she was doing fine after the Lasix."

"It's not just fluids in her lungs." Dr. Chavez explained, "Her chest X-ray looks bad. We might have to intubate her before the shift ends."

"Did you call her husband? What are the chances of a covid patient getting extubated and coming home to the family?" Maria asked him. "Maybe the husband will decide to let her be managed less aggressively. Would he consent to change her status? Make her a DNR?"

"She's only 44 years old. Her husband won't let her go easily without a fight", the doctor replied.

The low dose Metoprolol managed to bring her heart rate down and even with a second dose thankfully did not drop her blood pressure. Between nebulizer treatment every 2 hours, more Lasix dose, a higher level of Oxygen now at 80%, and a lot of prayers short of doing the rosary, Lina's vital signs stabilized. She watched her through the glass window as she's sleeping soundly now with another 0.25 mg of Ativan but her breathing was still labored. Maria thought to herself, there's another 20% more of oxygen if Lina would require 100% Hi-flow. I have another 2 hours before the end of my shift, what are the chances of Lina and I beating the odds. If she codes, it would be a horror show intubating a Covid patient.

The process is more complicated than a regular intubation on any patient. The risk and safety measures needed to put a tube down a covid patient's throat is horrendous. Endotracheal intubation is an 'aerosol generating procedure' with higher probability of transmitting the airborne respiratory particles than from coughing or sneezing. It creates a spray of infectious aerosols from the sputum and upper airway secretions of the patient, which has a high concentration of the virus. The PPE (personal protective equipment) consisting of impervious gown, hat, N95 mask, eye goggle, face shield may not fully protect the staff involved in the procedure.

Cecil walked in through the south entrance right beside room 301 as the clock strikes 7:00 am.

How was your night?" she asked.

Maria quipped back, "It's over!"

CHAPTER TWO

THE EARLY YEARS; THE BAD, THE GOOD & THE TRAGIC

Maria went home depleted and worn out. What just transpired in the past 12-hour shift triggered an avalanche of memories from the 20 years of her working at the BMT/ICU—a flashback of the good, the bad and the ugly. She remembered coming home after a shift, crying and distraught. She had to go to the emergency room even before her shift ended. She didn't want to but it's part of the protocol when you're stuck with a needle, contaminated or not. She was drawing the morning labs from the central line of an HIV positive patient when as she drew the needle out, it slipped and went through the gloves into her index finger. Horrified she came out of the room straight to the sink, squeezed her finger firmly, bleeding it profusely under a running hot water. "Holy shit!" she screamed inwardly.

"Maria what are you doing?" Mindy asked, "you've been in that sink for a long time."

"I've been stuck." Maria replied nervously.

"Oh no!", Mindy gasped. "I'll page the supervisor. Go down to the ED after you write an incident report", she added.

"I really don't want to. I still have to draw labs on my other patient. I'll be fine. I squeezed most of the blood right away."

"You have to go down." Mindy growled at her. "I'll cover your patients till the end of the shift. It's 5:30 now so it won't be for long. God knows how long you'll wait there till you're seen by a doctor."

Maria was triaged at the ED and waiting nervously with millions of fearful thoughts running through her mind. What if she gets infected with HIV? What if she loses her job just like the three ICU nurses that got exposed to the virus then later were terminated. How can she pay her mortgage? How can she support herself and her daughter? Wild thoughts running through her mind a thousand miles an hour. Then she heard a voice without sound.

"Fear not! God is with you always. Without fear, there is no danger, no harm. Fear is the magnet that attracts to you the one you fear the most. It is the cinder block that prevents the light that protects you to pour through."

She must have dozed off when she heard The ED nurse said, "a doctor will see you now". She led her to one of the small rooms where a harried young resident was looking at her chart.

"So, you've been stuck before?", he asked.

"Yeah, 5 years ago when I was working in a Dialysis unit, drawing blood from a hepatitis patient." Maria replied. "I got the Hepa vaccine, thankfully I didn't get the disease."

He wrote four prescriptions. Three were anti-viral drugs they call the 'cocktail' and one for Zofran, an anti-nausea medicine.

"I'll give you 3-day worth of supply then go to the employee health clinic after this. You need to be tested and be followed for a year. Before you go, I'll order blood tests for baseline labs", he added as he hurriedly left the room, jumping into the next.

She took the cocktail as soon as she got home. She only slept for 3 hours then started feeling nauseated. Even after taking Zofran, she was going to the bathroom every 15 minutes sick to her stomach vomiting whatever breakfast she had. She called the unit two hours before the shift. The secretary answered the phone.

"Hey can you tell the charge nurse I can't come to work tonight." Maria told the secretary, "I've been vomiting all day."

The second day of the anti-viral drugs, she took the Zofran every four hours, yet her body just would not agree with the drugs. She felt nauseous, dizzy and head achy. She wondered how HIV patients cope not only with the side effects of the drugs but the physiological, mental and emotional burdens of the disease, not to mention the stigma that comes with it.

Maria went to the employee health clinic after three days as instructed to. Another set of blood test was done.

"The preliminary result is negative and there's no viral load so far, but you have to take the cocktails as long as it's been prescribed." The nurse following her gladly told her, "I'll give you another 3-day supply.",

"I've only taken it for a day. I could not tolerate the side effects so I stopped taking it." Maria in all honesty could not lie.

The nurse was concerned, "You have to take the drugs, if you don't, you're taking a huge risk."

"I know", Maria replied, "but the side effects are killing me. I'll just wait for the result of the second test."

"Okay then", she said shaking her head in disapproval. "I'll call you as soon as the result is in and I will set you up for the next appointment. We have to check your blood every 2 weeks for a month then monthly for 6 months. There's the final test after a year. If it remains negative with no viral load, you are free."

And so, Maria lived in guarded, anxious moments for a year. But as the voice said to her in the Emergency room, "have no fear."

Even Yoda advised not to engage in fear, saying, 'It is the path to the dark side.' But working in the BMT/ICU unit for 20 years was treading on a multi-faceted dark side. Taking care of patients, seeing them suffer before they die, was just one facet. Another aspect was dealing with toxic co-workers and ego-inflated doctors who think they are the personification of God. And there's the nasty relatives that could blow you to smithereens. How can you not fear when you're immersed in the underworld of the BMT/ICU. Maria calls it the grand central of human suffering.

She was young and naïve when she first started working as a staff nurse at the BMT/ICU of St. Johnswart Hospital. Her heart bleeds at the sheer inhumane condition a patient goes through from the complications of radiation and chemotherapy. A person is healthy-looking when they first come in. They have to be, to withstand the rigorous treatment. They have to be cleared medically of any comorbidities or any physiological dysfunction. Their liver, lung, heart, renal functions have to be normal enough. And patients have to be physically fit to take the toxic barrage of chemo and radiation. After 5 days of conditioning with the lethal combination, the body starts to disintegrate in two to three-week time; hair falls down, bone marrow shuts down, mucous membranes slough off causing severe stomatitis that needs narcotic drips to offset the pain.

Patient has to be fed with total parenteral nutrition through a dedicated central line as they can't eat solid food with their mouths and throats scoured to perfect desquamation. Their immune system wiped out when the white blood cells are obliterated as well as the platelets and red cells requiring constant transfusions to prevent bleeding. They have to be protected from outside sources of infection by isolating them in reverse isolation. For a time while their counts are in nadir point, they have to live in a bubble of almost sterile environment of the laminar air flow room. It's a reverse isolation room where dirty air is filtered through a panel of HEPA filters, circulated inside and comes out through a 4x7 feet opening, where doors should have been but instead there's open portal in the left side of the see-through wall. There's no privacy except for a thick grey curtain hanging 3 feet from the plastic wall that can be controlled in a panel between the wall and the curtain.

Nurses were trained intensively to take care of these fragile patients; masking and gowning before entering a patient room; frequent handwashing before and after leaving the room; changing gloves as often as necessary when soiled while inside the isolation room. Patients were bathed with Hibiclens solution and instructed on stringent mouth care three times during the day with a nightly Gelkam routine as a Fluoride supplement. These practices have to be strictly adhered to prevent infection. At the start of the shift after report nurses have to scrub their hands for three minutes with a plastic bristle soaked in Hibiclens. In the Winter months, frequent handwashing turns Maria's hands into a rough, raw hide; a small sacrifice for the well-being of a patient, and nothing compared to what they go through after chemo and radiation.

One patient Lindy, a 24 years old girl diagnosed with ALL (acute lymphocytic leukemia), had 3rd degree burns from Ara-C. She hailed from a wealthy, privileged family living in an affluent suburb right outside of Boston. She was the picture of perfection when she first came in but there's a level of profundity lacking in her external beauty, the luster of which was skin deep. Her awareness of her not-so-ordinary beauty influenced her behavior and personality. She knows she's beautiful and that placed her above the ordinary-looking humans. But she's young. Her shortcomings could be excused by the folly of youth; a false sense of invincibility and pride that breeds arrogance. However, as the gods give it, the gods take it away.

Her induction chemotherapy after diagnosis consisted of the 7+3 regimen; 7 days of Ara-C (Cytarabine) infusion and 3 days of Daunorubicin. Cytarabine is an antimetabolite drug that disrupts cellular metabolism in cancer cells to prevent their growth and replication. It prevents further reproduction of leukemic cells by interfering in their DNA synthesis. However, it also affects the growth of normal cells in the skin breaking down DNA structures causing maculo-papular eruptions. She came in for HSCT (Hematopoietic stem cell transplant) and was conditioned with more Ara-C for 3 days. After a week into transplant, she developed cutaneous toxicity from the chemo drug; her arms, legs, back and chest have been badly seared with weeping blisters that have popped open. It took 3 hours to change the Xeroform dressing below layers of sterile gauze. She's practically mummified and as the old dressing was unrolled, the pain was so excruciating her screams were heart-wrenching and loud it could reach as far as New York city. Maria had to load her up with extra bolus of Fentanyl IV on top of the hourly rate, before she could start the dressing change.

"You're mean, you're mean, you're mean!!!" She screamed at Maria as she unpacked the old gauze on her legs, a new fist size blister just popped open oozing a golden, brown plasma from her excoriated skin.

"I'm sorry honey, I have to do this. If we don't change your dressing, your skin can get infected and that would be even worse."

"Mindy, can you give her an extra bolus. I got sterile gloves on." She yelled at Mindy who came when she heard the loud shrieks. "And give her a good dose of Ativan, she needs to be sedated."

Taking care of her day in and day out had exhausted Maria's sense of wonder how a human body can take so much blows from chemo and radiation. It's inhumane. Animals don't suffer this much, and if they're tortured, that's animal abuse.

Miraculously her skin got better slowly as her counts recovered after 6 weeks. However, she was traumatized, she would not speak or respond to any verbal cue or any kind of stimuli. A Neurologist was consulted but said nothing was wrong with her neurologically. She just stared into the vastness of space suspended between the talking dead and the living mute. A nasogastric tube was placed for her to receive oral medicines that's been crushed to get into her stomach.

Maria's been taking care of her consistently but one night she had a different assignment. She's glad and sad at the same time. She's glad to have a break from dressing changes, though it's not as much as it used to, but she's sad as she got attached and drawn to her silent world. She came by anyway to tell her she's with another patient but would gladly come check on her during the shift. No words came out but just rolled her eyes towards the ceiling.

Maria was in the break room when Mindy came in, sat beside her exasperated. "For the life of me I could not push any medicine through Lindy's tube. It's clogged. I warmed up the water, it didn't work. Can you help me?" Mindy asked Maria.

"Go get a can of coke and a 50cc syringe. I'll meet you in her room", she replied.

Mindy poured half of the coke into a paper cup and handed Maria the big syringe. Maria aspirated 40cc, then connected the tip of the syringe to the end of the nasogastric tube. She plunged the coke into the tube but felt a lot of resistance.

"This coke is too cold, give me some warm water to mix with it."

When Mindy came back Maria refreshed the syringe with the mixture of warmed up coke. She patiently pushed then pulled, pushing and pulling out the liquid... still not budging. The tube was stubbornly clogged.

"We might have to get a roto-rooter", Maria joked. She's getting frustrated now but remained hopeful. Maria was hunched over Lindy and noticed she's looking at her with a smirk on her face. Then all of a sudden, the patient blurted out.

"You look stupid!" she said to Maria with a bland expression.

Both Mindy and Maria broke out laughing hysterically. The mute now speaks, Maria giggling at her said.

"Thank you, Lindy. We're glad you're back. We thought for a while you've checked out."

Maria tried one more push and finally the solution went through.

"Yeehahh, success!" they both exclaimed.

"This would be a good coke commercial," Mindy remarked. "How did you learn this trick?", she added.

"I've watched too many video hacks on YouTube," Maria replied. "If it can unclog a toilet bowl, it can unclog a nasogastric tube, haha."

Satisfied, they both went on to take their break.

Mindy has been her close ally in the unit. They both started at the same time and went on the same orientation class together. They worked the evening shift and rotated to the night shift every other schedule. She would usually bring home cooked meal and they both take supper breaks together. She's very kind to her and has a gentle disposition, yet strong enough to stand up to any strong character in the workplace. In contrast Maria lacked the courage and unable to stick up to any conflict. She was born hiding from squabbles and had been hiding ever since. She just takes it, internalizes whatever it is that disturbs her emotional balance. One day, Mindy saw Maria came out of the staff's bathroom just outside the unit, her eyes red from crying.

"Are you okay Maria? Why are you crying?", Mindy asked, concerned. "Is it your HIV test?"

"No", she replied. "I'll be fine. I just have to chill for a minute."

"So, what happened? Tell me." She insisted. Maria hesitatingly answered, "Flambam yelled at me after I gave her report, told me I'm too lazy to hang a new bag and that I left her an empty IV bag. It's not even empty," she flailed her arms exasperated. "There's still 200 cc left and it's running to keep open at 20cc an hour."

"She's the lazy one," Mindy said. "She flabs around with her fake eyelashes and thinks herself the most flamboyant person in the world." She added, "And that's how she got her nickname."

The next day, as Flambam entered the report room, Mindy accosted her. "Hey Nightingale, who gives you the right to yell at anybody? You got the nerve to call Maria lazy when you left me a clogged NG tube. You can't crush the pills enough? Next time you bully my friend, you'll be in big trouble." She was just ignored except to throw at her an evil eye.

The BMT/ICU was staffed with mixed personalities. It's a tough group of nurses who bore the brunt of a challenging nursing practice. The charge nurse-Laura- has been there since it opened. She feels like she's the matriarch of the unit. She's laconic and laid back. Nothing fazed her even if the unit might be on fire. She took the role of the day charge nurse, though not official. In contrast, Marybeth, another senior nurse, was a dynamo. She's strong and unyielding even to people above her ranks. She yelled at interns and residents and didn't hesitate to question an order if it's not aligned with the well-being of the patient. Another personality, Bernadette, is the chain smoker who deals with stress with two- pack a day habit. She's scrawny as a single reed sticking out of a marshy ground. She doesn't eat, takes her 15-minute break down at the lobby sharing a smoke and stress stories with other employees.

The passive-aggressive joker, Brandon, was the male nurse as gay and bright as the Spring morning sun. He spins black humor out of the tragedy of the infirmed. Then there's Stacey, the blabbermouth. She walks fast, and talks faster with uncontrolled frenzy and wild abandon. She's all mouth on a walking stick spewing verbal diarrhea. Her monologue was littered with the f-word interspersed in every other sentence you couldn't make sense of what she's saying. But she's harmless. Underneath her verbal exuberance, she's warm and fuzzy with no ill will in her bones, unlike Flambam who's filled with self-righteous arrogance oozing out of her pores. She floated around in her pedestal. From a lofty perch of her towering ego, she sees herself perfect and higher than anybody, finding faults on everyone except herself. Her energetic signature has these written all over her; You didn't do this, you didn't do that, I'll report you to the nurse manager. She's condescending and arrogant.

Maria was the meek one. She's soft and sensitive but learned to toughen up through the years she has worked there. She's been taking care of this elegant lady, Mrs. Dean since her admission. She's classy, beautiful even without a single hair in her head. She changed her turban every day to cover her bald head with fine silk of royal colors- blue, purple and gold. Mindy said she's the wife of a real estate mogul in Boston.

"Have you met her husband?" she asked Maria.

"No, not yet', she replied.

"You're in for a treat, consider yourself forewarned", Mindy quipped. "He's here this evening for her transplant."

After a week of high dose chemotherapy and radiation, her entire immune system was wiped out. And when all her counts—platelets, white cells, red cells- were down to a dangerous level, a bone marrow transplant was performed to rescue her compromised immune function. It's not really a transplant in the usual sense but more of a transfusion of stem cells or bone marrow taken from a donor for allogeneic transplant. In her case it's autologous, taken from her own. The harvest from her iliac crest was minimal, 200cc compared to 500-600 cc of the usual yield for most people. The stem cells after it's been processed, are infused into the body via the circulatory system then finds its way into the bone marrow of the patient. It is equipped with a natural GPS - God Positioning system—that not one cell is lost along the way.

Maria has always been fascinated by the innate intelligence of the human body. How do those cells know where to go? The transplanted stem cells meander along the veins and arteries and with precision, lodge themselves in the myeloid tissues inside the bone. These progenitor cells will re-populate the marrow to produce fresh precursor blood cells that differentiate into white blood, red blood cells and platelets that sustain the human body. The procedure is life-giving to most, giving them a second chance like another birthday. Maria was glad to play a role in sustaining life however physically, emotionally, and mentally costly the procedure is to the patients and family, not to mention the enormous financial burden that comes with it. The transplant cost varies from 80,000 to 400,000 dollars depending on the case and complications that goes along with the process. For uncomplicated autologous transplant, average hospital length of stay varies between 3-6 weeks. For allogeneic cases, it could be 4 to 8 weeks and up to several months with severe complications.

Maria introduced herself to the husband sitting in the recliner beside the patient's bed, then addressed the lady in red turban.

"Hello Mrs. Dean, you must be excited, you're getting your cells back tonight."

She smiled weakly. Her marrow had been obliterated so her hematocrit was below normal. She's white as a ghost, paler than pale but assumes a proud bearing that material wealth usually brings. The husband, in his fifties, sat in the fullness of himself. He started fidgeting as if the chair can't contain him, not in the physical sense but in the expanded stature of his ego. He pushed it towards the wall to let Maria do the physical assessment on her wife. Something broke in the arm of the chair and he got upset and started throwing a tantrum.

"What kind of hospital is this? Chairs are broken, there are no Kleenex on her table, no plastic bag for her waste. Her table's messy!".

"I'm sorry sir I'll get someone to fix the chair". Maria said meekly and she left the room hastily. She thought... that's why Mindy told her she's in for a treat.

She came back to hang the pre-meds prior to the marrow infusion and hook her to the cardiac monitor. The husband was still fuming about something and throwing things around in the room like a three-year old having a tantrum.

"I'm not satisfied with how you take care of my wife." He told maria. "I expect a higher standard than what you are doing".

Maria asked herself, what have I done or haven't done? I barely started my shift. She would usually let the behavior slide but decided, not today. His sense of entitlement was way too big for her to swallow. For some reason she found the audacity to stare him in the eyes and stood up to him. She didn't care if he owns the whole freakin Boston city. Somehow, she got the courage to tell him off.

"I'm sorry for your frustrations sir, but if you feel your wife is not getting enough care, I suggest you hire a private duty nurse." She said it with a firm voice but her insides were trembling.

"How dare you say that to me." The husband was so livid. "I'm paying a lot of money on top of my donations I give to this hospital", he said fuming, the veins in his neck popping out.

"Where is your head nurse, I want to talk to her. I want another nurse to take care of my wife!"

Maria saw the charge nurse at the break room gobbling up on a piece of apple pie.

"Hey Laura can you change my assignment? I've been fired," she told her. "The husband doesn't like me taking care of his wife, Mrs. Dean. He says my service is below par, he wants another nurse. Can I switch with Brandon? I'll take my primary back", referring to the patient who called her stupid.

And so, at the middle of the evening shift, Maria and Brandon exchanged reports. Maria was glad she was fired by the Deans. The four hours remaining till the end of her shift was a walk in the park. Instead of the heavy dark cloud that hang about in the Dean's lair, she enjoyed the light energy vibe in Lindy's room. Her task was much lighter doing discharge teachings with Lindy, reviewing her home meds as well as the list of things she needs to be aware of when she gets home; a temperature over 100.5F, call the doctor; signs of bleeding, go to the ER and remember to wear a face mask when going out to public places. After her non-verbal stint she's talking up a storm, like she was given a new lease in life. Her skin has healed, her NG tube pulled out and now eating and drinking. There's a sense of buoyancy in her that she seemed lighter than a feather. The time period when she wouldn't say a word, she spent it immersed in a deep well of silence that refreshed and changed her. She was transformed. When she emerged from the dark void, there was in her an incredible sense of goodness. She's scheduled to go home in the next few days and that was one of the good things that happened in the underworld - the miracle on St. Johnswart.

Maria was off for a week, and when she came back, she was surprised to see a bulky guy wearing a white lab coat with a stethoscope draped around his neck standing right outside the unit. His right hip was bulging as if he's packing a metal. She walked past him ignoring the unusual sight and went straight to the nurses' report room.

"Hey Laura," she asked. "Who's that doctor standing right outside? He's just standing there like he's waiting for somebody?"

"He's no doctor." Laura replied laughing. "He's an undercover cop guarding the unit just in case Holly's husband comes back with more trouble."

"What?" Marias eyes popped out. "What happened while I was away?"

"We had an admission in room 21. Holly, a young newly married girl, 28 years old, from Maine diagnosed with Leukemia." Laura explained, "She's in bad shape, the doctors in Maine won't touch her so, she was transferred here for transplant. Her husband is a psycho."

"Really? We had some psycho personalities before, too," Maria remarked.

"Oh, this one tops them all." Laura said. "He's very unstable, came in drunk on the first day of her chemotherapy. He saw her retching her guts out after the Cytoxan. He came to the nurses' station wildly cussing. He accused the nurses and doctors of trying to kill his wife. He threatened to come back with a pistol and shoot all the staff that works here if something bad happens to his wife." Laura shuddered as she recalled the incident.

"I'm glad I missed the drama. Do I get her this evening?", Maria asked.

"No." she said. "You're too delicate for her, you can't handle the husband if he shows up. Smokestack will take her", referring to Bernadette, Bernie for short. Half of the staff calls her Bern, as in burn baby burn those lungs.

She looked at the assignment board and saw her name besides Mrs. Dean. "Oh no! I'd rather have the gunner's wife," Maria exclaimed.

Laura reassured her, "It's okay, the husband's not here. He's out of town for a week. Mrs. Dean actually asked for you, she wants to apologize for her husband's behavior."

Maria got report on Mrs. Dean and learned about what happened after she gave her up to Brandon for the remainder of the shift. The Fellow, who came to hang the marrow, spiked the plastic container so strongly that the pointy tip of the tubing pierced the bottom of the bag. Some of the precious content leaked out. The remaining cells transferred into a new sterile plastic pouch and transplanted to her while she slept.

"Did the husband saw it?", Maria had to ask.

"No." Stacey replied. "He went down to the lobby when the Fellow came up to hang her cells. When the husband came back, the cells were done, there's just a saline flush running through."

"How about Mrs. Dean?"

"She asked for another dose of Ativan, so she slept through the whole thing."

In the early years of transplantation, nurses weren't allowed to hang marrow cells. It's up to the Fellow to undertake the role of giving new life to the otherwise battered immune system. The BMT team from top to bottom starts with the Attending, then the Fellow, the residents, the Interns and at the lowest of the pecking order are the nurses. The Attending changes every month and depending on who's ruling the roost, the nurses are just the grave diggers.

Of her two patients, Maria went to see Mrs. Dean first to hang the last bag of the Potassium IV. She's awake, dignified looking in her silk robe and purple turban, yet she looked hollow inside. Physically she's here, but something inside her drifted off to distant realms. She's full of sorrow and regrets. Sadly, grief becomes her. The innermost glow has dimmed but a shadow of her beauty still remained.

"Hello Mrs. Dean, may I listen to your heart and lungs?" Maria started the conversation.

"Yes, you may. I'm glad to see you're my nurse this evening." She said weakly. "You know, it's been over three weeks since my transplant yet there are no cells growing. My bone marrow is still completely barren. Where do you think the cells went, Ithaca New York?" she jested.

Maria couldn't say, some of it dripped down the floor.

"Each person is different," Maria reassured her. "Sometimes it takes 2 to 6 weeks for the bone marrow to start making new cells. The doctors will give you GCSF, a growth factor to stimulate your marrow."

"I don't think I have more time to wait for my bone marrow to kick in." She gravely replied back. "I'll probably kick the dust before then. Healing has been a slow process ever since I got sick. What good is it to have all the money in the world if you don't have perfect health to enjoy it", she continued, "I realized now material wealth doesn't matter when death's door is staring you in the face. And I'm so sorry for how my husband had treated you."

Maria didn't have anything to say to that. And sometimes the best response is to just listen with a heart full of compassion. Mrs. Dean told her of her trips to Europe, Asia and South America, how she loved to travel, explored different cultures and see exotic places. They have wealth, privileges, honor and reputation, and in the face of an impending death, she found herself humbled. The threat of death looming in the horizon consumed all pride and prejudice. Maria didn't want to be rude but she said,

"I'll come back to hang your antibiotic, I just have to see my other patient."

She was in room 14 when Bertha, the aid popped her head.

"Maria, can you see the patient in room 21, she called twice and complaining of difficulty breathing."

"Where's Bernie?" she asked. "That's her patient.

"She went down for a smoke," she replied. "I told her when the patient called the first time but she said she'll be down for just a minute or two."

She proceeded to room 21 and saw the patient gasping for breath. She connected her quickly to the finger oximeter and saw her nailbeds bluer than blue, her oxygen saturation alarming at 76%, her heart rate 200/minute.

"Oh, shit! Call a code!", she yelled as she grabbed the oral airway taped behind the door of the closet where all the supplies were stored. She didn't have time to think how it should go down but intuitively slid the curved hollow plastic tube into her mouth with the tip touching the hard palate first then flip it sideways as it slid on her tongue down her throat, the patient gagging with the plastic piece. Mindy came in with the code cart.

"Good job Maria," she commented as she started bagging the patient while Maria hustled to connect her to the wires of the cardiac monitor. As Mindy pressed the Ambu bag the patient sounded like a rattlesnake on death throes. The code team arrived and took over the medical drama. Bernie strutted into the unit leisurely like walking along a silvery river under a moonlit night but gasped when she saw her patient being intubated.

Before the doctor could insert the Endotracheal tube down, a bunch of dead tissues sloughing off from the mucus membranes have to be suctioned out along with bloody secretions that clogged her airway.

"Give her a bag of platelets!", the doctor ordered. "And keep her sedated, she's bucking off the vent."

"Did anyone call her husband in Maine?", Laura asked the resident.

"I did, but he's not home." He replied. "The sister said he went hunting, won't be back for a few days."

"Oh dear, at least we have a few days before he'll be hunting us down when he comes," Laura remarked in jest but she couldn't be more prophetic.

The patient has been intubated for a week now but only the parents came to visit from Maine. The husband stayed away but when he came, he was so devastated nothing can control his anger. It was a mystery how he got past security at the lobby with a deadly weapon on him. He came barreling through the double doors of the unit. He started shooting randomly at the ceiling, the walls, the floors, with no specific target, no care, no conscience; just embroiled in a drunken act of mayhem born of deep anger. He was totally consumed by darkness. He splintered his pain with every bullet that came out from his gun. There was no God of Mercy, only his god of wrath eclipsing his mind and heart. With every gunshot a wave of fear rippled across the unit, prompting everyone to duck and hide where ever they can find safety. One last bang and then silence.

Maria was admitting a patient in room 17 when she heard the wild raucous. And where was the doctor/cop stationed outside the unit? He just happened to take a pee break in the staff's restroom by the elevator. When the Marshall and three blue uniformed men arrived, they found him in the stairwell, dead. He came to the unit unleashing his inner demons, lashing out not knowing where the bullet would land. In the end, he was certain where the last one would lodge - his brain. He shot himself with the last remaining bullet; one last act of a deeply unstable, deranged mind.

Chapter Three

A Kindred Spirit

The tragic incident made the administrators realized the hospital needed a strict visitor policy and metal detectors installed in all the entrances. The hospital, in all its highly reputable status, was reactionary at best. It took them awhile to institute a needleless system till after nurses have been stuck, three of whom got infected with HIV.

Maria was nearing her 6th month marker and soon due for another appointment at the employee health clinic. What if the result come back positive this time? What if she loses her job? Wild thoughts churned up incessantly in her mind as fear crept up in her like an unexpected visitor.

"Hush, hush, hush," she told herself. "Be still and know that God is mighty in you." That statement gave her comfort and she realized some thoughts are like intruding pests that sully the sanctity of her inner space. Even in deep meditation, they come uninvited. But just like guests, she learned to let them come and let them go. Her bedside clock broke her contemplation. She braced herself for another stint at the coal mine and hoped the natives won't be restless tonight as there's a big full moon rising up in the eastern horizon.

Maria had an admission in room 16, a 36 years old Tom McCormick from upstate New York. He's a software engineer newly diagnosed with AML (Acute myeloid leukemia). His blue eyes were deep-seated that reflected a mind that could fathom the mysteries of the Universe. He's soft and gentle in his demeanor. Maria sensed a nervousness in him as she explained the layout of the room.

"The closet beside the sink has the supplies- plastic spoon, forks paper cups as well as medical supplies. The panel on the left side of your bed has the controls for your curtains and window blinds."

Maria tried to make him feel at ease with a sense of humor, "Here Tom, you can change into this signature outfit before I get your height and weight." As she handed him the hospital gown and blue scrub pants.

"They are very stylish, opens in the back for reasons I have no clue of. Whoever designed this must be making millions of dollars by now."

He smiled wryly and disappeared in the bathroom. He's been there for quite some time. Maria was thinking maybe he's contemplating, 'should I stay or should I leave.'

When he came out, his face was full of dread. He looked like he's about to step into the dark side of the moon; uneasy, uncertain of the terrain he's about to tread on.

"Your suitcase is just outside. I'll bring your stuff in as soon as I wipe everything with disinfectant. Your clean clothes in the ziplock I can hand it to you now." Maria explained, "If you drop something on the floor, don't pick it up. Kick it out of the room, we'll disinfect it off before we can bring it inside."

She wasn't sure if Tom was taking it all in as he seemed distant, not interested in what she has to say.

The curtain outside the room parted as Mindy's head popped in.

"Hey Maria when you're done here, we'll take our break. I warmed up some moo goo gai pan." She added, "Tom, I'll bring you some if you want. You don't' have to start your BMT diet till tomorrow."

"Okay, thanks. Give me 10 minutes." Maria gracefully replied.

Before Maria headed to the break room, she took out the Poland spring bottle from her work bag in her locker and started gulping the tonic she brought from home.

"What's that liquid you're drinking? it looks like infected pee!" Mindy was curious. "It's my home remedy, and don't ask what it's made of. You'll cringe." She replied.

"Did you go for your 6th month follow up? What was the result of the test?"

"Yeah, I went last week. Thank God the lab test for HIV is still negative. This right here is my saving grace", she added as she finished drinking the 'infected pee'.

Up to this time she's still refusing to take the pharmaceutical combination of anti-viral drugs. Instead, she has been taking the alternative home-made cocktail every day since she got stuck.

Maria learned about the health benefits of garlic and ginger. She boiled the crushed garlic/ginger combo for 45 minutes. And when it's cooled down, she added apple cider vinegar with lemon in the mix. She hated the taste of it for the first few days but she forced herself to drink it. Adding honey to the cocktail made it more pleasing to the tastebuds. The tonic was her alternative treatment to the traditional, pharmaceutical route. She believed there's a holistic way to heal the body and she firmly believed in Hippocrates' saying, 'Let food be thy medicine and medicine be thy food.'

In the olden days garlic and ginger had been used to boost the immune system. Ginger has an anti-inflammatory quality to it and garlic has a potent anti-viral component that boosts T-cell production which is crucial to the body's fight against infection. Specifically, the cytotoxic T-Cells target cancer cells and directly kill infected cells compromised by viruses and bacteria. Research studies have shown that the plant compound found in garlic – allicin and diallyl sulfide – may help lower the levels of pro-inflammatory proteins like tumor necrosis factor-alpha (TNF-a) and Interleukin-6 (IL-6) that trigger inflammation.

Ginger compounds – gingerols and shogaols – inhibit inflammation and has a potent anti-microbial and anti-viral properties. Lemon is a known anti-oxidant which lowers the oxidative stress in the body that causes disease and dysfunction. The father of Medicine would be rolling in his grave to see how today's society has evolved into a pill-popping generation under the spell of profit- driven big pharma.

"By the way, Mindy what happened to Mrs. Dean in room 16?" Maria was curios.

"She coded the other night." She sadly replied back. "They couldn't bring her back after two hours of resuscitation, they put her on the vent for a short time. Finally, the husband let her go. She never engrafted even after all the Growth factor she got."

"I had a bad feeling about her last time I took care of her." Maria commented. "I think she knew her time was up."

Graft failure is one outcome of HSCT. Reportedly, there's 11% incidence of graft failure where the donor cells are absent in the blood and marrow of the recipient even after weeks of the procedure. The patients are left with pancytopenia making them susceptible to viral and bacterial infections. Some people come back for a second time when the 1st procedure failed. Mrs. dean didn't have the chance for a second one.

Others come for the third time. These people were brave enough to withstand the horrendous side effects. Like the myth of Sisyphus, the legend of toil and perseverance who was punished for cheating death, those who came for a third transplant, roll a heavy rock up the hill only to slip downward. Every time Sisyphus reaches the top, the rock would slide down then the cycle repeats again for eternal damnation. Some patients, by enduring the difficult process perhaps aim to cheat death or find meaning in the struggle. Either way, they have the wherewithal of resources - energy, family support and finances.

"How's your admission?" Mindy asked. "He's good-looking in most refined kind of way."

"Yeah. He's cute. He seemed reserve though. Politely stand offish. I sensed an invisible wall around him." Maria answered. "He looked at me with a blank stare while I'm explaining things to him as if he's not interested."

Laura came in the break room and said, "Hey girls sorry to interrupt the party but the Pharmacist's on the phone for you Maria. He already called twice while you were in room 16. And he's getting gnarly."

The pharmacist was in a bad mood.

"How many times do I have to call you guys to remind you to do your job. I need his height and weight now! And you haven't activated the chemo orders yet!" I'll be leaving in two hours. The night pharmacists don't do chemo."

'Hey chill, you'll pop a vein in your neck.' Maria wanted to tell him. Instead, she said, "I'll activate the chemo as soon as I find another nurse to cosign the orders. The height and weight are in the computer now." She said as she hurriedly typed into the computer the info written down on her scrubs.

The chemo doses are based on the BSA (basal surface area) calculated from the height and weight of the patient. Before it's administered to the patient the chemo orders had to be double checked by two nurses before activating them in the computer then approved by the pharmacist. If there's a discrepancy, the pharmacist calls the Attending. This double, triple checking of doses is necessary to make sure patients receive the right amount. It was unfortunate to hear about a couple of patients from a different institution who died of heart complications from an overdose of chemotherapy.

Most chemo protocols are straight forward but some requires a lot of marbles in your brain to calculate the doses which involve creatinine clearance. Majority of chemo drugs are renally toxic and some more so, which requires healthy functioning kidneys to excrete the metabolites, which are the byproducts of the drugs eliminated out of the body through the renal system.Maria went back to room 16 with two consent forms for Tom to sign. One for Central line placement, the other for blood administration. He's still awake going through the folder with all the BMT information in it.

"Hi Tom, you need to sign this before the anesthesiologist comes. He'll explain to you the procedure. You're scheduled for 9:00 am tomorrow. Don't eat or drink anything after 12:00 midnight." She added, "enjoy the night that you're free. Starting tomorrow you'll be hooked continuously on IV hydration during the chemo then the Tacrolimus line after that."

She explained to him what to expect for the next two weeks. She placed two urinals in the bathroom and a white plastic hat that fits in the back of the toilet bowl to collect the number two excrement.

"We measure your intake and output so use the urinal all the time."

He looked so overwhelmed and to make him feel better she told him,

"In the old days we insert a foley catheter before we start the chemo. We irrigate the bladder with continuous saline drip during the three days of Cytoxan. This flushes out the drugs from the body. Now we just ask you to pee on your own every two hours. And if your intake is more than your output, we force your kidneys to pee with a Lasix dose."

He winced at the thought of foley catheter.

"And you won't believe it," Maria continued, "Before, we bathe patients with warmed up sterile water from a 3 Liter bag using separate wash cloth for different parts of the body. Those days are gone. Now you can take a regular shower."

Maria brought his personal stuff in.

"These are all cleaned up." Placing his books and Cd's on the bedside table.

Two CDs are on meditation, four on the Beatles, and a collection of Secret Garden music. The books were on philosophy and spirituality.

"Do you like Wayne Dyer?" Maria asked, leafing through the book 'Your Sacred Self'.

"Yeah." He replied. "He's helped me go through some challenges in my life, both personal and work related."

"I like him, too." Said Maria, "I attended his seminar in Maui. I'm glad I went to see him before he died the same year."

"This one is good, too. I read it in one seating," she commented on Deepak Chopra's book- 'Quantum Healing'.

"Yeah, he's an excellent writer. He fuses medical Science with spirituality."

"Oh, this is heavy reading," Maria was impressed holding the book 'The Birth of Tragedy' by Nietzsche.

"No, not really," you just have to match his logic and level of understanding. He believed tragedy is the highest form of art. And he's right. There might be a 'metaphysical comfort' in human suffering."

"You're romanticizing pain and suffering. There's no way to romanticize the experience. However you look at it, it's a personal undertaking that one has to live through. Maybe a lighter attitude towards it would help bear it a little less heavy."

He was taken aback by her reply. He didn't expect it from her. He realized he found his match.

"Yeah, but there's a purpose to it."

She didn't answer but she thought to herself, 'what purpose would it serve except to keep the hospitals and big pharma viable. They seem to create more of it by generating side effects from the treatment itself.'

"The paradox of tragedy is that it could birth something beautiful and transcendental like a piece of art—a painting or a sculpture."

He's becoming more engaged now in the conversation.

"Oh, just like the Motel's song- 'only the lonely can play.'"

"Something like that."

Then he quoted Nietzsche, "To live is to suffer, to survive is to find some meaning in the suffering."

"Wow. You're a die-hard romanticist leaning towards the grimmer side of existence."

"At some point in our lives, we're just a fodder for the grim reaper."

"Okay, on that note, I'm just gonna take my leave now, you're getting morbid."

Maria saw a shadow of a smile on his face as he replied, "What do I do with this now?" asking Maria about the two urinals.

They started laughing like they've known each other for long.

The 36 years old man, who was clammed up earlier, now opened up like a book. Maria found the key to dissolve the invisible wall around him. She found a deep well of wisdom in him as they talked about the human conditions, how the seemingly random events in our lives are not random at all. She realized they share the same interest in spirituality, read the same books, enjoy the same music, and both subscribe to the philosophy of non-religion. In him she found a kindred spirit.

"Oh, wow. It's 10:45 already. My shift ends in 15 minutes," Maria gasped at how time flew. "I'll see you tomorrow. Hope you have a good sleep. Remember no food, no drink after 12 midnight"

"Okay, good night," he smiled at her with his deep-seated eyes, gone was the heavy cloud that hang over his head when he first came in.

Before she left, Maria put her name beside Tom's name on the white board where a list of the patients in the unit and the names of the doctors in the BMT team were written in black markers. She rarely signed up as primary nurse for any patient till now.

The next day, she came in excited to take care of Tom again but her assignment was different. She looked at the board. Her name beside Tom was gone.

"Hey Laura, I signed up as Tom's primary." She asked the charge nurse." Who erased my name on the board?"

"Brandon did. He wants him, he said you work the evening shift but he does the 12-hour day shift. You can have him when he's off or when he calls in sick." Laura was laughing.

Brandon calls in sick often, having regular diarrhea in the Winter months. But he comes back to work tanned from the Winter sun with wind burns on his face that tell tales of high-speed skiing. People knew he's not really sick when he calls but having fun with the elements in the ski slope of New Hampshire.

"Fine. I'm not even gonna fight him. But what gall he has!", she said resigned as she got report for her two patients, one was the girl from Maine, Holly. She was extubated after 2 weeks tied up to the ventilator. Her throat and esophagus started healing as the white blood cells start to come up but her marrow hasn't fully recovered yet. She's still needing blood and platelet transfusion every 2-3 days. Her liver enzymes were rising and her renal function doubling every day. She developed a generalized rash, the result of the skin biopsy of which revealed GVHD.

"Did she know her husband killed himself?" Maria asked the day nurse.

"No, the parents don't want her to know," she said.

"Does she ask why he's not visiting? What do they tell him?"

"Out on a long hunting trip." Said Stacey. "They do that in Maine you know, go hunting for weeks without coming home."

Maria went to her first after report and saw the Tacrolimus bottle almost empty. It runs 24 hours at a slow rate. The bottle change is usually at 2:00 pm. It's past its scheduled time and now there's not much left. She hurried to catch Stacey at the elevator.

"Stacey, the Tacro bottle is almost empty. There's no replacement on her med box."

"Fuck, I'm sorry I forgot to tell you. I called Pharmacy 3X. They said it will be here in the next round." She just shrugged her shoulders and off she went.

The med pump beeped, the glass bottle was bone dry. Maria saw the pharmacy aid dropping meds on the Suremed but there's no Tacrolimus in sight. She's getting frustrated, not knowing what to do.

"Where's that fuckrolimus bottle now", she's screaming inwards. She called the pharmacist with the intention of getting back at them. She wanted to even up and tell them to do their job but she just calmly said,

"I'm looking for the fuckrolimus bottle for my patient in room 21. The aid is here but he doesn't have it."

"It's been delivered hours ago," said the guy from Central pharmacy. "Ask him to look at other units, maybe it was dropped in the wrong place. Hey, is that the generic name for Tacrolimus? fuckrolimus?"

"It should be. It fucks up the kidneys." Maria laughed.

Laura heard her and commented, "Maria, I've never heard you swear before. Are you okay?"

"I'm good, thanks. I guess swearing is a release valve. I should do that more often like Stacey", she said.

Few minutes later the aid came back with the missing bottle, "it was on the other unit."

"Thank you." She said curtly. "I was about to hang my water bottle with infected pee." He looked at her with a face that says, 'you're weird.'

Before she went to see her other patient, Maria came to see Tom.

"Hey there. I'm not your nurse this evening. Brandon took over. He's gonna be your primary nurse. I just want to say hi. How do you feel with the new Hickman?"

"I'm sore but they gave me some pain medicine some time ago, but I don't like the side effects."

Tom set aside the book he's reading, flinching as he shifted his position. "These tubes sticking out from my chest is just bizarre. They look like big spaghetti noodles hanging out. Why do I need two double lumen Hickman lines for?" he asked.

"The right one usually is dedicated for your food line, the TPN (Total parenteral nutrition) that runs through one lumen, the other for Tacrolimus drip. They should be labeled so we don't draw blood from them. The left line is where we draw the morning labs and run your maintenance fluids as well as IV antibiotics. You might need a narcotic drip too, that's what the other lumen is for."

"What's Tacrolimus?", he asked like a child wondering whether it's good or bad for him.

"It's an immunosuppressive drug that lowers the risk of graft versus host disease, GVHD for short." Maria answered. "Who's your donor?" she asked.

"My twin sister," he replied. "I hope I don't get GVHD, we are 100 % matched."

"Even with perfect match, there's still that risk of rejection so the Tacrolimus just helps your body be much friendlier to your sister's stem cells so they don't attack your organs and tissues," Maria explained. "We start it as a continuous drip, but once you have enough therapeutic level in your system, the doctors switch it to a pill form."

Maria saw his face turned grim. "What's wrong?" she asked.

"I have to tell you. I don't really want to do this."

"Really? Whose decision is it for you to have the transplant?"

"My family, my wife."

Now Maria knew why he was noncommittal and guarded in his demeanor yesterday.

Brandon came as she was about to leave the room.

"Hey Maria, are you stealing my patient back?" he has the most irritating smirk on his face. Maria wanted to smack him but she ignored him and said goodbye to Tom.

Chapter Four

GVHD

Graft Versus Hot Disease

GVHD is a major complication of bone marrow transplant. Approximately 30-70% of marrow recipients develop rejection of the graft from the donor cells. The bone marrow or the stem cells recognize the environment it's been transplanted into (the host), as foreign and attacks the tissues and organs of the recipient. It's a hostile takeover of the territory, a vile betrayal of the hospitality given. It's similar to the theme of treachery in the Game of Thrones movie, where the Lannister clan, after dining and wedding the Stark family, turns around and attacks the unsuspecting hosts killing the step mother and brother of John Snow.

Similarly, the donor's stem cells enter the host's kingdom and wreaks unspeakable horror in various parts of the patient's body. It affects the lungs, the skin, eyes, the guts, and liver creating a slew of problems and pathological storm much darker than the original disease, the treatment of which aimed to cure. After the patient's own immune system is wiped out by conditioning protocols of radiation and high dose chemo, the donor's marrow takes over completely, setting up a new management of the immune system. The patient's blood type switches to that of the donor's, and even his allergies transferred into the host. The new management, though, might not be beneficial to the patient. It has a dark agenda that has to be tempered by an immunosuppressive drug.

That's where Tacrolimus comes in. It tempers the overactive immune function of the transplanted stem cells and acts as a mediator between the donor and the host to create balance and harmony in the body. It's the peace treaty between the warring warriors within the recipient who now hosts the donor's lymphocytes as well as his/her own immune cells. However, Tacrolimus has its own dark side.

After she left Tom, Maria went to see her patient in room 14, Maureen Finnegan. She's a 46 years old mother of three and a high school teacher from Andover, an affluent town North of Boston. She's into her 5th week of her transplant and developed GVHD of the liver. Her bilirubin was so high giving her the yellowest jaundice Maria has ever seen. Her legs were so swollen and her abdomen huge, it's a miracle she can still log her weight around to walk to the bathroom. Once she's up, she's okay to move about but shifting her position from lying down to sitting up, it pains Maria to see her struggle with much difficulty. She's still trying to maintain independence with daily task she needs to do-- mouth care 3x a day, Hibiclens sponge bath with little help and other activity that normal people just don't pay attention to, but to her it's a major struggle. She doesn't complain. She's rigorous with her mouth care not skipping a step, even the nightly Gelkam routine. Maria was awed by her strength and her ability to accept things as they are, resigned to her suffering as if, as she said, "my body is the cross I have to carry every day."

"Hi Maureen, I'll just come in for a quick assessment then come back to hang your 4 pm antibiotic. If you need to go to the bath room, I will walk you there before I go. I don't want you going by yourself."

"I'll manage, Maria. You're too small and too short to pry me out of this bed. How tall are you?"

"I'm five feet if my hair is permed, otherwise I'm 4'11" and a half. That half inch shrinks after a shower with my hair wet."

"You're funny. You make me laugh."

"Seriously, don't get up without any help. Do you need pain medicine? You're scowling with your eyebrows stitched together."

"I'm good for now," she said. "But if you bring me a red popsicle when you come back that would be wonderful."

She loved the cherry popsicle. It soothed her mouth which is getting better from the stomatitis, though not completely healed. She's off the Fentanyl drip, and even there's still lingering pain, she prefers the oral pain medicine as the IV medication makes her feel 'loopy'.

The high dose chemotherapy kills all quickly dividing cells like the cancer cells. Unfortunately, it doesn't discriminate the bad from the good. It also kills the healthy cells in the mucous membrane of the mouth as well as the hair follicles causing mucositis and alopecia. The transplant is like a rite of passage through a dark valley, where the patients pass through one challenge after another before they reach the finish line, the outcome of which is uncertain. Maureen has passed one obstacle as her mouth was healing but the graft was turning against her liver. Her GVHD was so advanced that she might need a new liver, as the doctors told her and her husband.

Maria gathered all the IV medication she needed for Maureen for the whole evening shift- Flagyl, Aztreonam, Acyclovir, Zofran and laid them out in the counter space right outside the room. The Micafungin for 4 pm was missing. She went back to the Suremed, rummaged the other patient's med box at the bottom of the big vault, but it's nowhere to be found.

"Where is my Mica-fucking-fungin?" she exasperatedly said out loud.

"Maria, are you okay?" Laura heard her. "You reached your swear quota for the day." She said laughing.

"I'm just missing drugs today," Maria replied. "First the Fuckrolimus, now the Mica-fucking-fungin, it's fucking up my day," she laughed as she's sounding more like Stacey. She was about to call Pharmacy when the aid rolled in with the IV medicine. She quickly grabbed it and proceeded to room 14, when the resident came up to her with a big sterile procedure kit.

"Are you ready?" he asked Maria.

"Ready for what?" she asked back.

He grabbed from his lab coat pocket a consent form signed by Maureen for a paracentesis and waved it on her face.

"Are you kidding me? That's fresh news to me." She said to the resident and turned to the charge nurse. "Laura, did you know about this?" she asked her.

"Yeah, why? Bernie didn't tell you?"

"No. She just said Maureen needs a bag of platelets and neglected to tell me why. Like Stacey she was in a hurry to get out."

"They're going on a double date." Mindy chimed in. "That's why Bernie took a 4-hour vacation time."

"They must be so excited to see their dates," Maria said, "They left things for me to sort out." She turned around and addressed the resident.

"You just have to wait till I give her the platelets. Her platelet is just 16K this morning, probably lower by now."

The resident was a little cocky. He said grudgingly, "You guys have to get your act together. Page me when the platelets are in." and walked away pissed off.

Maureen tolerated the procedure well. Maria gave her a dose of fentanyl IV before the paracentesis. Maureen held Maria's hands all throughout the procedure. A liter of fluid was taken out from her belly, now she doesn't look like a 9-month pregnant woman anymore. Maria was amazed how she can hold that much fluids in her belly. Her legs, though are still swollen. The doctor ordered six bags of albumin and a dose of Lasix. It's a pull and push strategy to remove fluids from the body; pulling them out of the 3rd space by virtue of osmosis. The albumin magnetizes and sucks the fluids out of the interstitial space into the circulatory system, then the Lasix pushes them out through the kidneys.

It worked because the next day, her legs were less swollen, her weight was down 3 kilograms. But it's all symptomatic management. After a few days, the fluids build up again in her abdomen and legs, just like the sea water flooding back the inlets in a shoreline. The paracentesis afforded Maureen a temporary respite but she's still facing a grave complication from the marrow transplant which requires a different organ transplant. Now she needs a new liver.

Another clinical manifestation of GVHD is when the donor's cells attack the recipient's skin. It's the most common complication after transplant that affects 60-80% of patients. There's degeneration of the basal cell layer of the skin as well as epithelial damage. Grading of skin GVH could be categorized in layman's term as mild, diffuse, worse and worst depending on the area of involvement. Worse is when the rash spreads over 50% of the body's surface area and worst is when there's generalized erythroderma with bullae formation.

Skin GVH alone without other organ involvement is less serious and can be managed by topical steroids and Tacrolimus ointments. For worst cases with a raging skin flare up, patient looks like a red lobster cooked to perfection. The doctors would order high dose of IV Methylprednisolone. Steroids are deemed a miracle drug but has its own side effects. Some developed steroid psychosis from it and weirdly enough, for one lady in room 12, it was exacerbated during full moons.

Nina, a 52 years old accountant who was so demure and proper when she first came in, developed strange behavior after receiving Methylprednisolone 2 milligrams of every kilogram of her weight per day for three days. After the steroid pulse, she seemed like she had a personality transplant as well. She would holler at the full moon, dance and twirl around in her bed with complete disregard of her own safety. She fell twice from her reclining chair jumping up and down, singing 'when the band go marching down.' At times she's combative that code gray had to be activated. You would think a couple of burly guys could tackle her easily but strangely enough, even with her small stature, she's very strong and hard to pin down. It was horrible to see her in 4 leather restraints as diminutive as she was.

Her skin care consisted of three different creams and ointments lathered all over body twice a day. Her rash, diagnosed as grade 3 Skin GVH from biopsy result, was diffused and extensive from face, arms, trunk to toes. The maculopapular rash is pruritic and painful. She needed to be pre-medicated with fentanyl IV before touching her skin. It took an hour to apply the topical treatment if she's cooperating, otherwise it took forever to cream her up.

Maria was taking care of her one day, and she's been off the IV steroids for a week, just being maintained on oral prednisone. Her rashes had toned down from angry, fiery pink to a pale brown hue. She's less confused now and begging Maria to release her from the two-point soft restraints that kept her from scratching her skin so hard it bled in some areas. Maria thought her mental status could be better. She thought wrong. As soon as she removed the soft restraints, she got up in the bed and started rotating clockwise with her IV lines wrapped around her. Brandon came and pleaded with her.

"Nina, sit down, you'll pull your Hickman out."

She looked at him fiercely. Waved her index finger on his face saying repeatedly, "Something's wrong with you, I know something's wrong with you. You're gay! Odd as the queer fish on a pond."

All these times that she has seen him around, she's been wondering what's wrong with him. It took a high dose of steroids for her to figure out he's gay. Mindy and Laura came by, gathered outside the open doorway asking Nina to calm down. Nina reveled in the attention she's getting. She escalated even more, twirling around like she's possessed by the devil. Good thing her head wasn't rotating independently separate in the opposite direction.

"Should we call code gray?" Laura said.

"Not yet," Maria replied. She turned to Mindy and whispered, "can you get sterile water? And put it in a cup."

"What for?" Mindy looked at her with furrowed eyebrows

"Just go." Maria had a devilish look on her face.

"What are you gonna do with it?" Mindy handed Maria the cup.

"Just watch."

She said to Nina jumping up and down, her IV lines wrapped around her.

"Nina, this is holy water from the holy city." She dipped her gloved hand in the cup and started whisking the water around Nina, below the bed, above the bedside table and back to Nina.

"In the name of the Holy Christ I command you Nina, be still."

Nina just ignored her and continued with her bouncing.

Maria repeated it two more times with a deep commanding voice this time.

"In the name of the Holy Christ I command, I demand you Nina be still, NOW!" Her voice carried a conviction of authority, she never knew she had. Nina stopped for a moment, looked at Maria with horror in her eyes but her expression changed to doubt and suspicion.

"Nahh, you just got that water from the sink. I saw you!", laughing like an old crazy witch then sat cross-legged on the bed, now chanting 'ommm'.

While Maria was doing the exorcism, Laura was pushing a good dose of the holy Ativan through her lines. Five minutes later Nina was out like a log. She slept for two days. When she woke up, she had no recollection of what she's been saying or doing. She was back to her old proper, demure self. After two weeks, her rashes got better, her mental status cleared up. Eventually she was discharged home to her family.

Maria's been working in the unit for two years now and she has shed some layers of her sensitive skin. She learned to toughen it out just as she has dealt with the tough new England Winter, though ruthless it may be. Working on the BMT/ICU Unit was as challenging as shoveling a 6-inch wet snow in a 20-degree windchill, with a 30-40 mile per hour wind gust howling at your face. It's brutal, but you have to face what's in front of you. You plow through the thick and thin of it. Boston strong. When strong is the only choice you have, you get stronger.

She came to work elated with some good news to tell Mindy, but she wasn't there. Her HIV test after one year came back negative. Her elation was dampened when she took report on her patient Maureen. She's dying. Her liver enzymes revealed advanced disease and family decided on no liver transplant. They made her a DNR. They would still continue on anti-GVH treatment.

"Hi Maureen, I'm here for you for this evening." Maria said, waving hi to her 3 kids and husband sitting in the folding chair, his face grave and heavy. "Enjoy the visit, let me know if you need anything."

"Can I have some popsicle?" asked the youngest one about 5 years old. "My mom says you have the best popsicle in the world!"

"Oh, sure! Come with me to the back room and we'll get a couple of them."

She took off her kiddie mask coming out of the room and they both went to the supply room where the freezer was located.

"You know, there's a popsicle genie in the freezer that when you ask her for something she'll give it to you."

"Hi genie," she said with pure innocence in front of the freezer. "I changed my mind I don't want popsicle now. Can I have my mom for Christmas instead?"

Maria almost broke down in tears in front of this beautiful child. Her chest tightened. She told herself holding her tears back, 'Maria, get hold of yourself. Be strong in front of this child. Let it flow, let it go!'

She took 3 popsicle and handed it to her.

"Christmas is not here yet, honey. You can have this popsies now. Here, give one to your brother and sister."

"Okay." She said and gladly skipped back to her mother's room.

Maureen's husband came out and hailed Maria before she went to her other patient.

"Maria, do you have time to talk?" he asked, taking off his face mask.

"Sure, we can go to the report room. There's nobody there right now."

He told her what the doctors have said during the family meeting.

"Maria, I was told she only has 2-3 months to live without liver transplant." And tears flowed down his cheeks. "I don't know what to do with the kids without her. I don't know what to do with myself when she's gone."

She was touched by this man's grief even while his wife is still alive. For a man he wasn't afraid to show his emotions in front of a stranger. She looked away so he couldn't see the revulsion in her face. Maria was utterly revulsed by the sheer arrogance of these doctors. Who are they to determine how long a patient shall live. They assume things far beyond the limitation of their knowledge. They usurp the power of the All-knowing Presence that lives in everyone.

"I'm so sorry to hear this, Jeff. But don't lose hope, miracles happen every day."

"Thanks Maria. I better go back to the room and let you get on with your work."

Brandon called in sick for the day, so Maria got to take care of Tom, who was in his second week of transplant. He's done with his chemo conditioning—3 days of Cytoxan, Ara-C, and Etoposide as well as radiation twice a day. She proceeded to his room. He was sitting in his bed retching and gagging, his face in front of the large brown rectangular basin used for bathing but also served as a puke bucket. The small emesis basin's not big enough to contain the spill-over of stomach contents.

"I'll hang your Zofran early, Tom" she said.

His eyes lit up when he saw Maria, sat up straight attempting to control what's coming out of his gut trying to look dignified in front of her.

"There goes my lunch." He said placing the basin on the bedside table.

"I'll give you IV Ativan after the Zofran." She said, taking the basin to the bathroom to be measured. The Ativan has magical qualities. It calms the nerves as well as squelch the threat of upchucking undigested food.

"Just the Zofran, Maria. I don't like narcotics. It dulls the mind and the senses." He said with firm determination. "I'm not being masochistic, but with pain and discomfort, at least I know I'm still alive."

He was watching her through the open bathroom door as she examined the contents in the bucket.

"Don't look at it too much, Maria" he said. "Some things are better flushed down the toilet." He's grinning now.

"No, I'm looking if there are pills in here so I could replace it." She said changing her gloves after washing the basin.

"Oh, like you would know which one is it." He's teasing her now and smiling with those beautiful eyes.

Maria went back to Maureen's room to hang her Mycophenolate, a strong anti-GVH drug. The family had left. She's resting in her recliner where she preferred to sleep. The bed was just too uncomfortable for her to lie in with her elephantine legs and massive belly. Reclined in the big boy padded chair, she looked happy and at peace. There was no suffering despite her condition she was in. Seeing her kids and husband sustained her, even just for a day. Maureen reminded Maria of the saying, 'pain might be inevitable in this life but suffering is optional'.

"Thanks for the popsicle, the kids enjoyed it." She opened her eyes as Maria came in.

"You have beautiful kids Maureen, especially the youngest one." She said, "I didn't mean to wake you up. I'll leave as soon as I hang your medicine."

Taking care of Maureen and Tom, Maria was suspended in a hanging bridge oscillating between two shades of stoicism, both remaining calm in the face of personal chaos. After Maureen she checked on how Tom was doing. He's dozing off with his ears plugged in to his CD playing the Secret Garden, the plastic case on his chest. He looked serene, engulfed in the soothing sound. What touches the heart may not be the same for everyone, but music for him carried the healing balm that salves his whole being in a deeper level. For Maureen, it was her loved ones that sustained her and gave her life and meaning.

With her two patients settled for now, Maria took her supper break alone in the back room behind the nurse's station when Laura joined in.

"Are you missing your lunch buddy?" She commented more than asking.

"Yeah. What's wrong with her? I thought she'll be here this evening. Is she sick?"

"No. She has some personal matters to attend to."

The aid popped in, "Maria, Tom is asking for you."

"Okay, tell him I'll be there in 5 minutes." She said swallowing the last piece of her sandwich.

"Hey, Tom you need something?" Maria asked as she piggybacked the Acyclovir to his main line.

"No, I just wanted to give you this," handing her the greatest hits album of the Secret Garden. "My sister brought it in the other day."

"Thank you. But that's for you."

"I have the same one. I asked my sister to get it for you."

Tom saw her teared up. "No big deal, Maria. I know you'll love it."

They both listened to the soft, lilting melody of the first track of the 'Dreamcatcher': 'Hear my silent prayer, heed my quiet call. When the dark and blue surround you, Step into my sight, look into the light. You will know that I have found you.' The whole Album basically evoked existential angst and the haunting music triggered an exchange of philosophical musings between them.

"Did you ever wonder why we're here?" he asked. "I don't mean here in this room, but why we're here on earth?"

"I don't know Tom, but that question is for Carl Jung or Nietzsche to answer." She added, "I do wonder sometimes why I became a nurse or who could I have been in this lifetime."

The music put her in a trance and a remembrance of her childhood came pouring in. She was pulled in a stream of consciousness with scenarios that Maria felt she was sucked into a vortex. She was looking at herself in a virtual screen with images of passing scenes:

My father was a fisherman, and growing up as a kid in a fishing village, I could have been a fish monger. Walking the pebbled beach, with a bucket full of uncertainties, rather than fish. Mongering fear and doubt to the hearts of the villagers, I could have been the best amongst the fish mongers.

Alternately, I could have walked the roads of Damascus as a silk trader, trading lies and deceit perfectly wrapped in a smooth satin fabric...trekking on my way to self-deception.

Or I could have been a carpet weaver in Tibet, trained in the craft of weaving intricate pattern of illusion; an adept at inter-twining threads of red, blue, yellow and gold into a geometry of Divine design. That's during the good days but on bad days, weaving each minute of every hour, each day of the week, each month of the year, creating a tapestry of illusory life.

But in this lifetime, I chose to be a nurse. Some kind of waitress waiting on people's pain and suffering, serving a platter of hope and healing. This, I chose not of my own design but a matter of economic persuasion.

Whatever I chose to do, where ever the setting is, however my motivations are... the fact remains that my life, my role, my time is but a short pause in Someone's eternal musing.

"Maria to earth, earth where's Maria?" Tom snapped his finger at her. "Where did you go? You left me here for a minute."

"You were asking why we're here? I think we are here to play a role, different roles lifetime after lifetime until we finally figure out who we really are." She said, "and we have to play along with different types of people."

"My father used to say, there are two types of people in the world—the winners and the losers." He said, "but I think it's not just black and white. There are different shades of black, various shades of white and different shades of gray."

"Yeah, there are skimmers and there are skippers." She added. "The skimmers just skim the surface of their own lives. They don't look beneath the water to see how seaweeds live."

"Or how the corals thrive." He added, "and the skippers hop and skip their own problems, not facing them till it bites them in the arse."

"The skippers are the best escape artist. They binge on Netflix, if not alcohol or drugs to escape painful stuff." Maria said with one person in mind- her husband.

"There are wingers, too, without wings." She added. "They wing their way through without a thought of what they do. They just do it."

"They should be called Nikers. Like the Nike ad—just do it." He laughed. "You know what's worst, "he asked.

"No, what?"

"The schemers. They plot and plan their lives at the expense of others. They steam roll anyone that gets in the way."

"There are the scammers, too." Maria added. "They are the low-lest of the low, the scavengers preying on gullible minds."

"On the higher end of the human spectrum," she said, "there's the space holders."

"Yeah, I think they are the noble ones." Tom replied back. "They are generous enough to hold space in their lives for peace, and love and light and pour it out into the world."

It's strange how they finish off their train of thoughts as if they shared the One Mind, both connected to the same Source.

"Should we create a game? - name that type." Maria joked. "Forget Carl Jung's way of classifying people. This fits the generation of today.

"And who and what are you?" Tom asked.

"I may be all three-- a skimmer, a skipper, a winger, but never a schemer, nor a scammer?"

"You don't scheme to get what you want?"

"No. God gives me everything I need when I need it." Maria replied with conviction. "If I don't get what I want, then it's not for me."

At this point, the curtain outside parted and the aid peeked in, "Maria, Maureen wants some pain medicine."

She went to room 14 with a vial of fentanyl and a card for Maureen. She's of Irish lineage so Maria didn't feel out of place giving her a card with a photo of the sacred heart of Jesus.

"Maureen, the Fentanyl will help you sleep through the night," she said. "And I hope you don't find me presumptuous if I give you this."

"Oh, thank you. I love it!" she said reading what's at the back of the card.

"There are two versions of the mantra and both affirmations, when uttered intensely can be a powerful healing tool."

The first affirmation reads:

In the name of my God I AM Presence, in the power and authority of my Holy Christ Self, I decree, I can heal myself through Christ who gives me strength and power. I can heal myself in the love of my Divine mother. I can heal myself in the sacred fire of St. Germain. I have faith in myself and the Wisdom, the Power, the Love who created me.

The second one reads:

IN the name of Jesus the Christ, I decree: Today I am healed, I am whole, I am complete for within me is the healing Presence of Divine Light that never fails and I am one with my God I am Presence. I AM, I AM, I AM. By all God's love, by all God's Light, I am healed. And so it is, done!

"This is just so beautiful, Maria. Thank you."

"Good night, Maureen, hope you have a restful sleep. It is your strong faith that can heal you."

"Good night, dear, be safe on your way home."

The following day, Brandon came to work. Bernie on seeing him hollered, "Hey Brandon, how's your diarrhea?"

"Better, thanks." He replied. "How's your lungs? You still got two of them?" The rest of the staff within earshot, laughed as the two bantered at each other.

Maria had the guy in room 17, a 62 years old professor of Economics at UMass Boston with an impressive array of academic credentials. He had two Masters and a PhD. He's cultured by virtue of lifelong educational attainment but turned surly as a result of frequent trips to the bathroom. His transplant course was complicated by acute gut GVH. He puts out 4 to 5 liters of liquid diarrhea a day, and it's bloody, and stunk to high heavens. She wouldn't be examining the contents prior to flushing it.

"Hello professor Downs," Maria greeted him. "Can I get you anything before I gown up?"

"Just call me Gerard, or Jerry," he said gruffly, running to the bathroom trailing foul smelling maroon stool on the floor with visible specks of his innards. "Get me a dose of Morphine. This pain is killing me."

"Okay, I'll be right back."

Graft Versus Host disease has three phases. The first phase starts during the first week of admission when the patient is conditioned with high dose chemotherapy and radiation. Both cause tissue damage, which triggers the release of inflammatory cytokines. Cytokines are proteins that regulate the inflammatory process, which is the body's reaction to injury or infection. They are also released when there's a threat of tissue damage caused by radiation and chemotherapy. This first phase called Afferent phase initiates the body into billowing symptoms of bodily dysfunction – nausea, vomiting, diarrhea.

The second phase- the Efferent phase- happens after transplant when the donor T-cells interacts with the host's immune cells called APC (antigen presenting cells) causing further inflammation as more cytokines are released by the activated donor T-cells. The activation of the donor's T-cells stokes up the fire of inflammation started in the first stage.

T-cells or T lymphocytes are a subtype of the white blood cells that helps the body fight infection as well as destroy the body's own cells that are either infected by viruses or have become cancerous.

The 3rd phase- the effector phase- is when the recipient's T cells are activated and react to the donor's antigens. This results in the migration of the cytotoxic T cells and natural killer cells where they target organs causing further tissue damage leading to organ dysfunction. Natural killer cells (NK-cells) are type of immune cells that kills both infected and cancerous cells. The activation of NK cells in the host is accompanied by secretion of pro-inflammatory cytokines which even drive up the inflammatory process.

The immune system, of which the white blood cells are part of, is a vast intelligent network of checks and balances that sustains the body and protects it from invaders like bacteria, viruses and toxins. It is the first line of defense on the look-out for threats. This protective mechanism is made up of the skin, the spleen, thymus, lymphatic system and the bone marrow that produces platelets, red blood and white blood cells. It has an innate intelligence that maintains order in the body to maintain health and well-being.

The process of BMT/HSCT brings chaos and disorder in an otherwise orderly Universe that is inherent in the human body. GVHD is the perfect out-picturing of the law of entropy brought about by three different players: first, chemo and radiation launch the 1st attack. Second, the donor's T-cells stir up the peace by establishing dominance and control, and thirdly, the recipient's immune cells launching a strike back attack like soldiers who have gone rogue. The transplant process typifies a random decline into a greater state of disorder.

In gut GVH, the intestinal villi - tiny hair-like structures - that line the intestinal tract responsible for absorbing fluids and nutrients, are destroyed triggering a widespread inflammation in the gastro-intestinal system. This brings about apoptosis or programmed cell death to rid the body of unhealthy cells devitalized by chemo and radiation. The symptoms start with nausea and vomiting. It progresses to severe abdominal pain caused by a widespread inflammation of the alimentary canal. Then there's the secretory diarrhea that turns bloody with the sloughing off of the intestines.

For some patients, the diarrhea is mild with 500 cc to a liter a day. For Jerry, with grade four gut GVH, it was an endless trip to the bathroom, putting out over 4-5 liters in a day. Maria gets exhausted watching him go up and down his bed to the bathroom and oftentimes with a trail of his entrails.

"Jerry, I'll get you a bedside commode so you don't have to go all the way to the bathroom."

"No, thank you." He said, and he got gnarly. "Don't deprive me of my dignity Maria. I like to stay private in the loo."

"Okay. Let me know if this dose of Morphine is enough. If not, I'll give you more." She said, "the doctor ordered a range."

"Give me the whole thing, don't skimp on me now."

"I'll give you a dose of Ativan, for your nausea. The combination of the two drugs might make you unsteady on your feet. I don't want you, scuba diving on the floor." In your own filth, she added in her mind but instead she said,

"These two will give you a good night sleep."

"Are you kidding me? Sleep and diarrhea don't go together. You want me to sleep and shit in bed at the same time?"

"Hopefully the diarrhea will slow down after this first dose of steroids." She said as he administered the wonder drug through his lines.

The doctor ordered him a pulse of high dose Methylprednisolone, 10 mg/kg every day for three days. Maria said a little prayer to the steroids god to spare him from psychosis, otherwise it would be a shitshow. Literally.

Chapter Five

Anatomy of a Divine Romance

It's the middle of ski season. Brandon was in his usual winter retreat, and today he didn't show up for work. Stacey took care of Tom in the morning shift.

"Brandon's having diarrhea, again. I hope he's not spilling brown liquid in the mountains in Vermont. Are you ready to get report on Tom?" Stacey asked Maria.

"Sure. Give me a sec to put away my bag and jacket."

It's 15 minutes before 3 pm but Stacey was eager to get home. Maria wondered if she has a follow up date with the same guy.

She finished her report by saying, "Sorry, I didn't have time to change his Hickman dressing. Could you do that for me? If not, I'll do it tomorrow if Brandon doesn't show up."

"Sure, I'll do it."

Maria could have said, 'It doesn't take 15 minutes to change the dressing. You can do that now if you wanted to.' But she didn't.

"Oh, he needs a bag of platelets, too. They increased the parameters above 50 thousand because of his hematuria."

"He's bleeding in his urine now?"

"Yeah, and he's passing out clots, big clots and it hurts him to pee." Stacey added.

She went to the supply room to get the dressing kit but she couldn't get herself to start her shift. She's still revving up from the argument she had with her husband before she left for work. She sat on the stepping stool and started crying.

"Maria, what's wrong?" Mindy asked as she walked in.

"I just got a terrible headache. I should have called in sick." She said wiping her tears away. "I'll be okay."

"I have Advil in my bag. But I have a feeling it's not gonna take care of your headach e.""I gotta go change Tom's dressing," she was evading Mindy, and she headed to room 16.

"Hi Tom, can I come in to change your dressing? I'm your nurse this evening."

"Sure Maria. I'm glad to see you." His eyes perked up when he saw her.

She was fumbling with the last tape as she finished the dressing, when she felt Tom's hands rested on her left forearm, touching her ever so gently. She looked at him looking at her intently. There's so much tenderness in his eyes that Maria melted. All the heavy feelings she was carrying dissolved like a mist dissipating in the warmth of the morning sun. She tried to avoid his gaze as she was feeling uneasy.

"Maria, look at me. Let it go. It will be okay." Tom sensed what's going on in her internal world and knew the misery she's feeling. Is she so transparent? She asked herself. Or is there a deeper connection between them that they have felt the first time they've met.

She looked at him and realized what a beautiful encounter to look at someone's eyes looking at you through the eyes of a loving God that knows no imperfection; just savoring the sweet essence of you. Their eyes locked, triggering a soul remembrance. At that moment they were two ancient time travelers intersecting at this point in time from across lifetimes, spanning multiple dimensions. They were not just two ships passing in the night but two divine lovers meeting once again in the darkest points of their lives. His blue eyes reflected the depths of the ocean and the vastness of interstellar space. Like a reflecting pool, Maria saw in those deep eyes the multiple lives they shared in past incarnations in Tibet, Persia and Damascus. The scenarios she thought she was imagining when she was in a trance were not from her wild imagination but a vague recall of her past lives; as a fish monger in the Persian Gulf, a carpet weaver in Tibet, a silk trader in Damascus. They were two old souls coming together once again, this time they're in the opposite side of the fence; her being the nurse, and him being the patient. They are both married with kids, and both were miserable in their married life.

Tom was still holding his arm when the aid, Bertha peeked through the curtain.

"Maria, your other patient is calling." She said, looking at them weird, her mind going off with wild conjectures.

"Tell professor Downs, I'll be with him in five minutes, I just have to empty the urinals while I'm in here so you don't have to gown up. Or do you want to come in to do this?"

She hastily disappeared to avoid the chore.

The steroids had worked its magic on Jerry. His stool output had markedly decreased and his disposition much better.

"Hi Jerry, you looked much better now. What can I get you before I come in?""You mean less grouchy," he said. "Can you get me one of those pain medicine?"

"Are you still having abdominal cramps?

"Not as bad, but I just like the feeling after you push that Morphine."

"Sure. I'll be back." Maria thought, at least he's honest.

"Oh, Maria, get me some Ativan, too, and my regular oxycodone."

Jerry came in with a long-standing prescription of oxycodone for his old injury sustained while he was in the military. He built up tolerance to it that his dose has been escalating.

Mindy was in the Suremed taking meds for her patient.

"Thanks for the Advil, Mindy, I missed you the other week we were supposed to work together. Where have you been?" Maria was glad she's working with her this evening.

"I missed you too, Maria. I'll tell you later, my patient- Holly is not doing well." She said hurriedly, as she headed to her room.

Maria gathered all the meds for Jerry for the whole shift and as she laid them in the counter outside the room.

"You're so organized Maria," Jerry commented as he watched her.

"Thanks Jerry. I have your morphine and I'm not skimping this time. Don't hesitate to ask when it's due. There's more where it came from." She was joking with a hint of sarcasm. They both knew he's starting to like the drug a lot more than what it's supposed to do.

"We're defying the principles of economics here. There is no scarcity in the pharmaceutical bin especially in the drug business." She added.

"Did you know I am a professor in Economics?"

"Yeah. Were you still teaching before you got sick?"

"Of course, and I'm hoping to get back when I get out of here." He added, "You're very smart Maria, you should pursue your Master's degree."

"I actually applied at your school. I thought I wanted to take my masters in Biotechnology, but I was denied admission."

"Did you interview with the department?"

"Yeah, the guy was so condescending. He said to me, 'So, you're a nurse. Nurses don't use their brain much and you want to take Biotechnology?'"

"Bastard! I hope he doesn't get sick and ends up here like I do. You nurses are pretty smart."

"It wasn't for me, and it wasn't the right time."

"Don't let that asshole derail your aspirations for higher education." He said, "there are other schools out there and much better."

"Thank you, sir. I'll take you up on that, and if you don't need anything else, I'll take my supper break now. Call if you need something, I'll be at the back room."

Mindy and Maria took their break to catch up on things.

"I was worried about you when you didn't come to work last time. Were you sick?" Maria asked.

"No. I had to see my divorce lawyer."

"Oh, I'm sorry to hear that, Mindy. I'm also having problems with my marriage. We actually had a fight before I came to work."

"That's why you were crying when I saw you in the supply room?"

"Yeah. I hate to bring my personal life to work and vice versa, but sometimes it just spills over. You're the only one I can tell stuff to."

"Me, too. I don't trust anybody here. They wag their tongues like dogs wag their tails." Mindy said. "Oh, my blood is here for Holly. Can you check this with me?" as the aid came in with a bag of red cells for her patient.

The staff of the BMT/ICU was an amalgam of personalities that, although they're pretty much a caring group of people, there's a dark side to their goodness. Nurses take in blows from different corners -- from doctors, relatives, patients - and one way to vent it out is by lashing at each other. The accumulated stress in the work place was expressed laterally with back stabbing and petty outbursts. Maria liked most of them and she admired their dedication to patient care, however, she stayed away from the dense energy that hang about in the unit when certain personalities were around.

Maria went home that night hoping to avoid further confrontation with her husband. She's been married 14 years and she had enough of marital discord. He's been spending a lot of time at his friend's house, four to five times in a week, coming home drunk and wasted in a state of Smirnoff. She stuck with the marriage for her daughter's sake. He's not physically abusive but the emotional abuse was worse than any physical harm. She felt alone without any emotional connection with him. It still hurts her to think of the time when she got sick and passed out in the bathroom floor. She didn't know how long she was out, but when she regained her consciousness, she couldn't open her eyes. Her legs felt like lead, couldn't move them even if she tried to. When she opened her eyes, she found herself wedged between the toilet bowl and the vanity table. She heard the TV in the living room and called him for help. He knew what happened but just chose to ignore her. Maria somehow found the strength to crawl out of the bathroom towards her bedroom.

Entangled in the stress of challenging work situations and the reality of a dysfunctional married life, Maria learned how to cope by going inwards. Yoga and meditation were her paths to staying sane. She took refuge in spiritual books. That, and she slept for the days when she was not working. Sleep was her escape hatch from her outer reality.

Maria wanted out even in the early years of their married life. She was so fed up she took off, went skiing in New Hampshire with her two friends on the day of their 7th year wedding anniversary. She remembered the feeling of freedom and fun going down the hill despite her not knowing how to ski. She took lessons while her two friends were already doing runs on the intermediate slope. After three lessons on the kiddie slope, she thought she's ready for the ski lift. She went with her two friends up the mountain riding the chair lift and looking down the evergreens on the sides of the trail, Maria felt exhilarated in a good way.

They were nearing the top of the mountain approaching the station where two attendants were on the lookout.

"Okay Maria, get ready to jump." Her friend warned her.

"Will this lift stop?" she asked.

"No. It will go around the station and go back down, so you have to jump when it gets to the landing."

"Here we go. Jump Maria!" And the two left her still sitting on the moving chairlift.

"What? Jump where?" She was expecting a flat surface but the snowy ground was uneven with big bumps of crackly ice on the landing ground.

"Holy crap, I don't think I can. I'll just go back down on this darn lift."

"Come on Maria, jump. You can do it." Her friends yelling at her as the conveyor gearing to turn around from the top of the mountain to go back down.

She summoned enough courage and in one sweeping moment, she jumped and landed upright with her boots and skis still intact on her feet. Her friends were laughing at her but she felt a little pride to have accomplished such a small feat.

"Remember, pizza to stop. Parallel skis to accelerate downhill." Her friend said.

"Got it." She said as both took off in the whiteness of the mountain.

She stood on top of the trail enjoying the view, told herself, "I can do this."

A small voice said, "you can't. You'll fall to your death."

A different voice whispered, "God already has gone forward before your fear. He has paved the way for you! Just have fun on your way down the trail."

Maria took a whiff of the frigid air and stood at the precipice of self-discovery. Going down the mountain would either win her a small victory or a small death. But she learned fear is just an illusion. It's not real. What's real is the beauty in front of her; the pristine white snow, the towering Cypress trees on the side, and the scenic silhouette of New Hampshire mountains in the distance. She firmly held onto her ski poles and with one push, she let go of fear. Now she's held in a bubble of excitement, gliding down, zigzagging in the snowy trail.

Challenge accepted, she beamed to herself. It was petrifying and thrilling at the same time as cold air whipped on her face. She felt care-less and free. She had never felt more alive in a long time. But as she accelerated down the hill, she couldn't control her momentum.

'Pizza to stop', her instructor said. 'Turn your skis from parallel position to a pizza pie formation.'

Her sense of exhilaration turned to panic as the skis crisscrossed forming an X. She lost her balance, landed on her bum with her legs perpendicular to her torso, her skis up on the air. And that's how she skied halfway down the mountain, luckily without one broken bone.

She saw her two friends heading back to the lift, summoned her again to go with them.

"Maria, ready for another round?"

"No thanks. I'm good for now. I'll save my courage for another trip." She headed to the coffee shop to wait for them there. A little bruised but she felt proud of her small victory and celebrated it with a hot cup of coco. She was grateful that she remained whole and bones intact after the fall. An hour later, the two friends came, obviously exhilarated and had their fill of the Winter thrill.

Her reverie was broken by the sound of the side door opening. Her husband walked in smelling like the whole brewery.

"What are you doing here?" Maria asked with contempt. "I put all your clothes out on the front steps. Go live with your friend. You spend most of your time with them anyway, even on your work days."

"You forgot my underwear. It's not in the plastic bag," he laughed in a drunken state and passed out in the living room couch.

The next day Maria went to work with a heavy heart still burdened by the squabble she had with her husband. She lightened up when she learned about the positive turn of events in Maureen's condition. She's fully engrafted and her bone marrow's fully functioning, producing adequate white cells, platelets and red blood cells that she's requiring less frequent transfusions. Her liver function tests were slowly coming down, her liver decreasing in size, and her abdomen less bulky.

"It's really a miracle how she turned around after the doctors had given her a death sentence." Laura finished her report saying, "I hope we get a lot of miracles like that."

"I'm so glad for her kids and the husband." Maria replied.

Maureen was an exceptional woman. She plowed through her suffering with dignity and fortitude. With firm determination to heal and be with her family for Christmas, she meditated on the picture of the sacred Heart and saying the affirmations three times a day incorporating it with her daily routine. Her fervor, in a short period of time, shifted her reality from infirmity to a world of healing and transformation. With strong faith and intense devotion, in her daily communion with the sacred heart, she developed a relationship with her Maker. She raised her consciousness and entered into a transcendental romance with the Divine. She had given all her worries, all fears and totally surrendered herself to a loving, merciful Presence that no matter what happens, she's okay with it. She asked herself, "In the presence of GOD, what is there to fear?" Nothing!

When she prayed, she didn't beg to be healed. Instead, her prayer was an act of communion with the Source. In stillness and reverence, she merged with the benevolent father. And in that quiet union, her miracle was born as she opened herself to grace. Her heart aligned with the Sacred Heart, her life became a living prayer, a continuous connection to God through gratitude, love and surrender.

Maria went to her first after report.

"Hi, Maureen. I'm so happy to hear the good news. Your family must be excited. You're going home in time for Christmas."

"Yeah, thanks to you I was able to heal myself. You gave me the gift of healing."

"I'm so proud of you. I can't take credit for it. It's your faith and the love of your family that are the most powerful forces."

Miracles are manifestations of Divine Love. It doesn't follow a linear path, nor does it wait. It just happens spontaneously and instantaneously defying logic. It is governed by quantum laws and requires nothing but a shift in perspective from a limited 3rd dimensional thinking. For it to manifest, there has to be an unwavering trust without a shred of doubt in a Higher Power and not so much dependence in Medical Science which is symptomatic management at best.

Maureen, with her unequivocal trust, emerged from the shadows of doom to a world of transcendent light where miracles happen. She was sustained by the most powerful force in the Universe – love, and the prayers of her family especially the little one who believed in the popsicle genie in all her innocence. Love is the true medicine. Her family's love was the only medicine she needed to heal.

Brandon was out again so Tom was assigned to Maria. She tried to change her assignment, "Can I have Holly instead of Tom?"

"Bernie is here, and she is her primary." Laura replied. "Besides, Tom is asking for you. He likes you more than Brandon."

And that's how the rumors got started. That, and the aid, Bertha blabbering, telling people that she saw Tom and Maria kissing. From an innocent gesture of Tom holding Maria's arm for a brief moment, the incident got blown out of proportion to Tom kissing Maria. It's like the story about a snake killed by a man, the size of which got bigger and bigger as the story is passed on from one person to another. No wonder every time she walked into the unit, she's the object of demeaning looks from Stacey, Bernie, Flambam and Brandon.

Maria got report for Tom from Stacey. In his 3rd week of transplant he developed hemorrhagic cystitis, a complication from Cytoxan which requires keeping his platelet parameter higher than the usual 20,000. He was passing out blood clots in his urine and having bladder spasms. He was having frequent and painful urination that a foley catheter inserted during the cystogram was decided to be left in place.

Cytoxan has a metabolite called Acrolein, a byproduct of the drug's metabolism that is filtered by the kidneys then accumulated in the bladder. It's a corrosive substance that causes ulceration of the bladder wall exposing the underlying blood vessels resulting to hematuria. It basically breaks down the DNA structure as the cell membranes are disintegrated in an inflammatory response to the toxic metabolite. Acrolein is also a major component in cigarette smoke as well as charred meats. Smoking and eating overly charred barbecued meats are two risk factors and a double jeopardy to one's health. The metabolite from an alkylating drug like Cytoxan potentially brings about pyroptosis which is cell death by necrosis in the urothelium of the bladder.

The aid brought in the platelets for Tom. She handed it to maria without looking at her, like she's guilty of something.

"Can you take Tom's vital signs?" Maria asked her. "And tell him I'll hang his platelets as soon as I checked this with another nurse."

She ran off without saying anything, like a dog with its tail between her legs.

"Hey, Tom. Your platelets are here. I have to disconnect you from your other line to run this through." Maria said trying to avoid eye contact with him.

He was sleepy from the premeds Stacey gave him before she left, but he sat up in his bed as Maria walked in.

"I hate this catheter. Can you take it out?"

"You need it, Tom. The blood clots in your bladder block your urethra, keeping the urine from flowing out, and gets your bladder distended."

He started flinching, "the bladder spasms are killing me."

"I'll page the intern to order you something for it."

Maria was with Maureen doing discharge teachings when the intern called back.

"Hey, did you page me?"

"Yes. Tom 's having bladder spasms, can you order Ditropan for him?"

"I'm not sure about that. I'll ask my resident."

Five minutes later, a short plump resident rolled in asking, "Who's the nurse asking for Ditropan?" with a tone of her voice demanding to know who dares tell them what to order.

"That's me. I'm taking care of Tom and he's bladder spasm is bad." Maria said, "I wonder if you can order Ditropan to control the spasms."

"I'm not gonna order it." she said firmly staking her authority over her. "I'll order him Morphine for the pain."

"He doesn't like narcotics, that's why maybe you'd consider Ditropan first."

"Do you know that it causes urinary retention?" she's getting riled up.

"Do you know he has a foley catheter? By virtue of gravity the urine flows down into the bag." She said in a small voice.

She got so flustered, "how dare you tell me what to do. You're just a nurse, good at menial tasks. Go empty that foley catheter."

Maria must have bruised her ego, probably insulted her medical license.

"I'm just asking if you would consider it first."

"I'm the doctor here. You don't tell me what to do. I have more knowledge than you." she said, her red face turning pale white as if she's seen a ghost when she saw Marybeth approaching. At that point she walked away.

Maria's getting perturbed herself, she had never been in a collision course with anybody before, except that time with Mrs. Dean's husband. She can taste her gall coming up her throat. She's not comfortable with confrontation. She has to compose herself before she goes back to her patients.

Marybeth heard the whole thing.

"Hey, Maria don't let her bother you. She's got some issues with Napoleonic complex. She has to assert her authority to compensate for being short." She said laughing. "I had a blow out with her, too when she was just an intern."

"Oh? That's why she left in a hurry. She's scared of you, she turned pale when she saw you, haha."

"I'll page the attending. He'll order the Ditropan." She added.

Marybeth was one of the most senior nurses in the unit. She's feisty, doesn't back down in any conflict or clashes of viewpoints. Her knowledge base and clinical experience was strong and commands respect from her peers as well as some doctors. She's stoic and calm for the most part but don't trigger her. Her outburst could be lethal.

"Maria, I talked with the attending. He's ordering Ditropan and he wants Tom to get started on bladder irrigation." She said, "And that's how you deal with residents, you go over their heads to the top."

"His catheter needs to be changed to a 3-way foley. Can you do it for me?" she asked.

"Why? Are you squeamish, you haven't seen a penis before?" she was laughing.

"I'm not squeamish. I'm just not good enough doing it."

"I'm just teasing you, Maria. Go get the supplies and I'll meet you in his room."

Marybeth was explaining what they're going to do when Maria came in with the catheter and a 3 Liter bag of saline hanging on a pole. Tom looked uncomfortable his eyes got so big when Marybeth unfurled the catheter.

"Whoahh! That's a garden hose, much bigger than what I have now."-

"It's a 3-way foley, the saline flows through one lumen into your bladder while the urine empties out through the other one. The third lumen is for the air to inflate the balloon so the catheter doesn't slide out." Maybeth explained. "I have a urojet. It's a local anesthetic to numb your penis."

"You'll feel much better after the clots are flushed out." Maria added.

Marybeth must have done this a thousand times in her nursing career, as she inserted the tube easily, and she's not squeamish. She then attached the saline line to one of the ports, opened the roller clamp wide open and a deeper shade of rose -pink urine with clots flowed freely from out of the red sea.

"You can titrate the flow Maria once the urine gets clear."

"Okay, thank you Marybeth."

"No problem, you owe me your first-born son." She joked as she stepped out of the room.

"Is she that tough?" Tom asked. "She practically manhandled me!"

"She looks tough, some interns are afraid of her. But she's good tough. Working here must have toughened her. She's been here since the unit opened."

The following day, Maria was hoping to have Maureen again for her assignment but she had the professor in room 17. He's much improved with less stool output which dwindled to 400-500cc a day. The steroids had abated the inflammation in his gut and lessened his abdominal cramps but he's still asking for pain medicine. He liked the euphoric feeling of IV Morphine and now he's chasing a temporary high, romancing the drug, drawing him to a blooming love affair with the opioid. He's drawn to a different kind of divine romance, although far from being divine. He gets sourly when he can't have his fix.

"What do I have to do to get pain medicine here?" she told Maria when she answered his call.

"It's not time yet, Jerry. You got the full dose 2 hours ago. It's ordered every 4 hours as needed."

"Well, then you just have to page the doctor to get me an extra dose." He said getting belligerent.

"Okay, I'll try."

The intern ordered a x1 extra dose in addition to the prn order. She gave it to him and an hour later Jerry was calling again.

"Maria, how much did you give me? It didn't work."

"He ordered half of the usual. Wait another hour and you'll get the full dose."

"I want it now and I want the full dose!" he's getting ornery and hostile.

Exasperated, Maria asked Marybeth, "What shall I do?" He wants more Morphine."

"You know what you should do?"

"What?" Maria asked desperately.

"Give him a dose of IV Ativan to calm him down. Then follow it with a push of sterile saline but chill the syringe first in the refrigerator for 5 minutes."

"Really? Would it work?"

"Push it fast. The chilled saline will give him the same rush."

"I'll give you my second born son if this works." And so, Maria learned a trick that she hoped she will never do again.

"You don't even have a son." Marybeth laughed, "you only have one daughter."

Ten minutes later, she asked Maria, "how did it go?"

"I guess it worked, he's flat out snoring now."

Brandon was on vacation so she took care of Tom. He's getting used to the foley despite his aversion to it. Third week into his transplant, his marrow was staring to grow new cells sprouting like the flowers in the early spring. He's getting discouraged, though with the onset of hematuria but Maria's presence uplifted him.

"Maria, how can you do that? Constantly emptying the bag below and replacing the bag above." he asked watching as she dumped the pink-colored urine in the toilet bowl.

"This is not my first rodeo I was trained to do this when I worked at a TURP unit in Texas. All I do the whole shift is empty red urine, like endlessly bailing water out of a sinking ship."

"What's a TURP?"

"Transurethral Resection of the Prostate. I didn't last long in the unit. I had to bail out, no pun intended." She laughed.

The sound of her laughter buoyed him. He found the courage to tell her how he felt about her.

"Can I tell you something Maria? I hope you won't get mad."

"What is it? You need nausea medicine?"

"I'm drawn to you like a magnet. Tell me you feel the same. I don't know why, I felt like I've known you before in some past lives."

Maria couldn't say anything. She, too, felt the spark between them even on the day they've met for the first time. And the spark grew into a flame of attraction. But it's not physical, rather, it came from much deeper than skin and bones. It's a quantum entanglement from a soul level that dates back to the birth of time, crossing multiple lifetimes. She used to dread coming to work but now with Tom in the unit, she's excited to drive to the hospital to see him even for a brief moment.

"Maria, can you say something?"

She turned her face away so he couldn't see the tears flowing down and pooled behind her mask. That was the only confirmation Tom needed. There was no questioning of what might be ambiguous in her feelings, for there was no ambiguity in the fullness of her heart. Now she let her guards down. She looked at him, his eyes fiery and penetrating, dissolving the façade she tried to hide behind. In his eyes she saw the expanse of misery he had traversed in multiple lives and the heights of passion he pursued in the past. Now, there's neither passion nor misery, just the flame of divine love, a fire consuming all desires and what's left in the ashes was the purity of Higher love.

Maria could not tear her gaze away from his eyes. She was drawn to the depths of his soul and in turn he was mesmerized by the crystalline purity he saw in her. There was magnetic attraction born not of the flesh but of the spirit. There's synergy between them, both uplifting each other to a higher octave beyond human understanding. It's not an affair of the heart but of the soul, a divine romance which is ephemeral like the gossamer wings of a butterfly that fleets from rose to rose to the butterfly bush that knows no time. It's not everlasting but infinite in the ever-present moment of the here and now. There is no judgment, no expectation, nor attachment...just pure bliss in the delicate gentle flight of love's longing for that effervescent feeling of loving someone deeply and being loved in the same way. In that timeless moment, they reached the heights of heaven without even trying. They felt an addiction to a natural high, an exhilarating speed of love's momentum taking them both to the highest peak. It's an orgasmic sensation of spiritual connection; the tingling of the spine even without touching and the electrifying feeling permeating every cell of their beings. Their hearts were full, filled to overflowing.

From cloud nine the two lovers were brought down to earth by the voice through the intercom.

"Maria, Jerry is asking for more pain medicine." Bertha's voice came through the intercom. At least, she's not sneaking around this time.

"Tell him I'll be there in two minutes." She said scrambling to finish emptying more pee from the foley bag.

"What took you so long? I need more pain medicine. This cramps just won't go away." Jerry demanded when he saw her.

"You're not the only patient here, Jerry." Maria was getting miffed by his demanding attitude. "I'm giving you the full dose of Morphine and Ativan so you can sleep through the night."

"What about my oxycodone? It's ordered every four hours."

I'll give it to you in 15 minutes, it's not due yet."

"What's 15 minutes, I need it now!"

Maria went back to the Suremed and grabbed all the narcotics he's ordered for. Sixty mg. Of oxycodone, one mg of Xanax and Ambien for sleep.

"This guy is a walking pharmacy. I'd be dead taking this much oxycodone." She mumbled to herself.

She went back to the room and found him chatting lively on the phone. This was the guy supposedly in pain.

"Here's your oxycodone, Jerry." She opened the 12 tablets of 5 mg. each and handed it to him in a medicine cup.

He counted the pills one by one, "I'm missing one oxy."

"Count it again, I wouldn't stiff you Jerry or I'll be fired."

"Oh, sorry. It fell on my lap. Is my Xanax here?"

"Yes sir. And your Ambien."

Maria felt like a drug pusher, with a license at least. She's not comfortable giving drugs to feed the addiction but it's not up to her to judge the rightness or wrongness of it. Patient wants it, it's ordered by the doctors, so it's legal. But legal doesn't make it right.

Maria went home mulling on the contrasting picture of Jerry's dependence on Morphine and Tom's refusal to use narcotics for his discomfort. What makes one crave for the high of the narcotics to avoid the pain while others chose to stay with the discomfort and let the strength of his willpower dissolve it. Maybe it all comes down to the type of person they are - a Skipper and a Niker.

Chapter Six

Nightmare After Nightmare

Maria couldn't sleep right away when she got home at midnight. She did her meditation for an hour to decompress from the stress of the previous shift. In her alpha state she saw herself walking on a deserted road dimly lit by the waxing moon. She was carrying a heavy bucket full of fish to be sold to the village folks. Her father, a fisherman comes home from night trawling and asks her daughter to peddle the night's catch. She knew she was dreaming and dreams don't make sense. They're just jumbled pieces of random scenes that confound the mind as to its meaning.

In her dream, her path took a turn away from the village center towards the shoreline of an ancient place as she heard a soft voice whispered in the wind, "Come to the water's edge."

Then her dream turned to a nightmare as two dogs, one black the other white, appeared on her path. The black dog was menacing, angry looking with its fangs exposed ready to pounce. The white dog seemed gentle and non-threatening as it stared at her fiercely. She stood frozen in her tracks. She's afraid of dogs, the phobia of which started after she was bitten at an early age. As she turned around to avoid the mean looking dog, they started chasing her as she ran as fast as she could, her bucket she dropped behind. She told herself,

"This is not real, It's just a lucid nightmare. I can control how this end."

As she reached the water's edge, she stopped running and faced the two canines now a yard away from her. She faced them with strong stance and told them, "Stop, you have no power over me."

The white dog turned around and walked away, the other came closer. The dog's face morphed into a man's face, that of her husband.

"Maria, wake up. It's 12:30 pm. Aren't you going to get ready for work?" her husband's face on hers as she woke up from the nightmare and thought, this is the real nightmare she'd rather not face.

"I'm not working this evening." She replied still feeling exhausted from the chase.

"Oh, okay. Get up anyway and eat something. I made you breakfast, it's lunch now."

She almost fell from her bed lying down. That's a surprise, she wondered what brought the change of heart.

"Are you not working?" She asked wondering why he's home on a Monday.

"I took the day off. Maybe later we could talk."

"Thanks for breakfast, I'm just gonna walk around the arboretum."

After eating she grabbed her jacket and headed to her wooded bliss a few miles from her home. Winter should be winding down and soon the crocus and daffodils would be coming out after the last frost of the season. She thought with anticipation of the heady scent of Spring flowers especially the lilacs. The arboretum was her sanctuary. She felt sheltered by the trees and finds a loving, comforting Presence in the towering hickories. They have ears that listened to her woes and worries. She's more connected to them than her husband.

From the arboretum she drove to Jamaica Pond. The still water of the pond has a way of absorbing her troubles and cares. On placid days when the breeze stands still, a sheet of glass appears on top to mirror the white clouds above. She's amazed at how it's never the same at any given moment. It is a dynamic eco-system for ducks, kids, lovers and loners. With the Southwesterly wind blowing, the watering hole appeared to her as if engaged in an ecstatic fusion of wind and water creating tiny ripples that washed away her sins.

Maria walked towards where the mighty oak trees rise over the rolling hills on the South end of the pond. She's awed at how they survived since the 18th century through the wicked blizzards of New England. This year, the Winter season was unforgiving. Nor'easter came and went, four in a row, one each week. Now, in the front steps of Spring, Winter is not yet dead. This gave her a frozen resolve. She, too, like these ancient trees shall weather the storms in her life.

It was chilly to walk around farther so she drove to Chinatown to see a psychic medium.

"There's a heavy cloud above you." She said right away as she walked in. "I know why you're here."

Maria told her of her dreams and asked her what it meant.

"The dogs represent your fears. You running away means, you're not facing it and the heavy bucket is the heavy load you're carrying. The shoreline is your gateway where you can unload your cares and worries over to the ocean. Let the tide carry them off to the depths to be washed away." She added, "the other dog that turned around is your other love. You're not meant to be together in this lifetime." She finished her reading but still her eyes were glued to the violet crystal ball in front of her.

"Wait, I see a storm brewing in your horizon, both in your personal life as well as work. But fear not, you'll overcome them all. You have powerful guides and angels around you."

Maria already knew the symbolism of her dreams. She didn't have to pay 100$ for a psychic to tell her that, but she wanted a second opinion. Her mom used to say, "if the load you're carrying is getting too heavy, put it down."

She went home and found her husband waiting. She smelled Johny Walker all over him.

"I answered the phone the other day," he started. "It's from a lawyer, a divorce lawyer. Maria, are you filing for a divorce?"

She looked at him squarely in the face. This was the nightmare she was most afraid of, the confrontation she's not ready to deal with. She hoped the lawyer could have been more subtle.

"I think we already reached the end of the rope where there's nothing to hang on to."

"We could get another rope, a brand new one." He genuinely thought he could change her mind. "We could start all over again. I'll check myself into a rehab."

"You've done that twice already. Both times you didn't bother to join the 12-steps program."

"How about our daughter? She's only eleven."

"We'll share joint custody." She didn't say, she's the reason I hang on for so long.

"Maria, we've been married 14 years. You used to say it would be nice to grow old together."

"Growing old together happy, not alone in the marriage. You spent more time with your friend than me and your daughter."

He didn't want to hear the truth. He'd rather skip the existential dread, a typical 'skipper', he stomped off, left the house and went to his friend's house.

Divorce was the bitter pill she had to swallow. She's been simmering in the bitterness of her relationship it's choking the life out of her. Brewing in the cauldron of marital discomfort for a long time, she's ready to jump off like the proverbial frog getting used to the warm water till it reaches the boiling point. She's chained to his dark valleys while his soul was tethered to the bottles of gin and vodka. His world fogged up by the fumes of alcohol, he didn't realize the effect of it on his family. It not only diminished his own worth but made Maria felt abandoned and depreciated with his outbursts when drunk and when he's not fueled up, his apathy drives a wedge between them.

Maria knew she's not perfect either. She has her own faults magnified by the acrimonious relationship. Her heart shriveled, locked up in rancor. She longed for a time when love was pure and wholesome. She has to get out of this unholy matrimony before she drowns. To her, in love there's no depreciating others, rather, love enhances the value of the beloved and make them whole and complete. Unless one truly loves another, relationships are mere playgrounds for ego dynamics and power trips.

Going back to work after being off for 3 days, she was in for more nightmares. She was glad Jerry was gone. He was discharged to a drug rehab center. Tom was still hooked to the bladder irrigation, though his hematuria was less.

Maria got off the elevator as Mindy came out from the other adjoining metal box.

"Maria, the nurse manager was looking for you the other day." Mindy was particularly disturbed. "I heard rumors about you and Tom having an affair?"

"What?" That's crazy. How did that happen?" she was flabbergasted.

"We'll talk later. We'll go down to the cafeteria on our breaktime." She said and proceeded to get report for her two patients.

Maria had Holly this time. She's fully engrafted with her bone marrow producing mature healthy cells but she developed respiratory distress syndrome with persistent dry cough and dyspnea on exertion. She's dependent on oxygen, and she's hovering on the brink of being re-intubated again. She's on 100% Hi-flow mask with her oxygen saturation fluctuating 90-92%. She was intubated the first time for obstructive reasons; dead tissues sloughing off from her throat and blood pooling from her oral mucositis obstructing her airway. Her throat and mouth had healed since then but her lungs were brewing up a different cytokine storm.

"She's scheduled for lung biopsy tomorrow." Bernie said in report, her eyes looking at her as if she's got scarlet letter A tattooed on her forehead.

Maria went to get Holly's nebulizer from the Suremed and saw Brandon and Stacey standing by the nurses' station next to the Suremed machine. They were chatting about something with malicious undertones. As soon as they saw Maria, they scattered away like pesky flies, but not before they throw evil looks at her that seemed like daggers in her heart. She kept her cool. She's here to work, she told herself. She gathered everything she needed for the shift and stayed away from them.

"Hello Holly, I have your Tessalon Perles, your cough medicine." Maria asked, "What would you like to drink?"

"Just a little water please." She said in between coughing fits as she went into violent bronchospasm. "The nebulizer treatment would help relax your airway." Maria wished she had a much better way to ease her coughing and a magic wand to dispel the evil causes of disease.

Even before the result of the lung biopsy, the doctors already knew Holly's transplant was complicated by lung GVHD. Her PFT's (pulmonary function test) showed a restrictive lung disorder alongside her progressive respiratory symptoms. The high dose chemotherapy and radiation caused an injury to the lung tissues which triggered an immune response from bioactive compounds such as pro-fibrotic cytokines, the main culprit in the inflammatory process in her lungs. These renegade chemicals induce stiffening and fibrosis in the pulmonary parenchyma. Another biologically active compound that contribute to the storm of inflammation are the leukotrienes. Derived from Leukocytes, they are the Darth Vader of the immune system. Upregulated in acute respiratory syndrome and allergic reactions, leukotrienes bring about tightening of the airway muscles as well as excess mucus production.

There are natural remedies that block the production of Leukotrienes like aloe vera, Boswellia, black cumin, ginger, garcinia, green tea. Other chemical compounds like quercetin, found in many fruits and vegetables such as onions, kale, capers-- has an anti-inflammatory and anti-histamine effect. Natural flavonoids like Galangin and Chrysin found in honey has an anti-viral, anti-microbial effect as well as help reduce inflammation. Capsaicin found in peppers and curcumin also help block the production of Leukotrienes.

But Maria can't possibly say to Holly, "Here's green tea and garcinia, take it three times a day and be forever healed." She'll be shunned as she was already.

Maria replaced Holly's Hi-flow mask with the nebulizer mask connected to a separate oxygen flow meter. Even for a brief moment of switching masks, her saturation drops below 90's, her coughing exacerbated.

"Maria, are you okay to take a break now?" Mindy's head popped in.

"Not yet," she replied. "I'll come out after I settle her down with this nebulizer treatment. Oh, can you get her a liquid morphine? I think she's ordered for it."

The Tessalon Perles wasn't strong enough to quiet down her cough. Maria was torn listening to her incessant coughing, that her own chest hurt for her. Holly's airway was restricted by the inflammation in her bronchus and lungs that it pained her to breathe. She could see her abdominal and intercostal muscles working hard as she struggled to inhale the Montelukast aerosol treatment. She held her hands just to reassure her, she's not alone in her suffering.

Mindy came back with the morphine and a bag of platelets."I've double checked this already with Laura, so it's ready to go. The doctors want her platelet count buffed up before her lung biopsy tomorrow." She added, "Bernie called from her car, she said she forgot to chart down the premeds she gave her before she left."

"Thank you, I'll run these platelets through then we could go down to the cafeteria."

The liquid morphine helped sooth Holly's throat and lessened her coughing and with the Benadryl pre- med, she finally settled down for a nap.

Mindy saw Laura by the nurses' station.

"Hey Laura, we didn't bring food today. Maria and I are going down to the cafeteria. Can you watch my patients?"

"Can you ask Marybeth to watch Maria's patients?" she added.

"Sure, enjoy your break girls. Bring me some apple pie when you get back." Laura replied.

The two nurses found a quiet secluded section in the cafeteria away from the rest of the hospital employees, where they can exchange the latest news hot from the gossip press.

"Have you read your work e-mail yet?" Mindy asked her.

"No, not yet. Why?"

"The nurse manager, when I saw her the other day told me she sent you an e-mail. I don't know why she particularly had chosen me to tell you."

"Maybe because she knows we're friends." Maria replied. "So, what's this rumor about me and Tom having an affair? Who started it, do you know?"

"Bertha told the unit gangsters--Brandon, Bernie, Flambam and Stacey-- she saw you and Tom kissing. And they all went to the Nurse Manager and said you're having a liaison with Tom."

Maria almost choked on her French fries.

"What? That's beyond ridiculous! How can I have an affair with a man 7 years my junior, tied up to a bladder irrigation, pissing out the red sea?" her face turned red with dismay and anger mixed up to a boiling point. She felt sick to her stomach.

"You have to confront them, Maria. Brandon, Stacey and Bernie, they all want you fired."

"I can't get fired now. I'm going through a divorce."

"That's why you have to clear your name. Did you read the e-mail from the NM?" She said looking at her watch, "Oh, look at the time, we have to go back. I have to hang an antibiotic on my patient."

"Yeah, she wants to see me at her office tomorrow before I come to work."

They went back to the unit, Maria feeling so drained and weak from the false accusations she was just slapped with. The rest of the shift, there was a heavy cloud hanging over her head and she wanted to cry but she had to hold herself. This, too, shall pass, she told herself. For now, she had to stay strong. This was another nightmare she had to deal with and what the psychic was referring to.

She drove home to find her husband drunk as usual, waiting for her. He started his gibberish slurred speech wanting to talk about their marriage.

"Not now. I'm so tired and wiped out, I just want to sleep." And she slammed her bedroom door to his face.

She put a pillow on her face and let out a muffled scream, her tight chest about to explode. She cried so hard to let the pressure out, but the pressure kept rising as she sunk deeper into the abyss of pain. She found herself free-falling into the depths of the oceanic trench. Her world turned dark and she's at the bottom of the pit being buried alive by the dirt and rocks being thrown at her. She's living a nightmare, one after another. Her marriage in shambles, she might be losing her job, and her co-workers putting her in shame. Now she understands the saying, 'when it rains it pours.' She trembled and sobbed for hours and there's no stopping the dammed-up tears she held for so long.

The next day she went to work early and went straight to the nurse manager's office. She was waiting for her.

"Maria, I just want to hear your side of the story. If it's true, you know it's grounds for termination."

"It's not true. I swear on my father's grave." She said calmly. "I don't know how the rumor got started but if Bertha is here, I would like to ask her to be here, too."

She dialed the unit's phone number, asked the secretary to ask Bertha to come in to her office. She's working the day shift so she's still around.

Bertha's eyes grew big when she saw Maria. She wasn't expecting her there. She thought it was for something else, like somebody complaining she's not doing her job.

Maria wanted to scratch her eyes, pluck it out of her vile socket but she remained poised and collected.

"Bertha, in all honesty can you tell the Nurse Manager what exactly did you see that day?" Maria asked her with firm voice.

She started squirming, trying to justify the lie she's started. She can't look at Maria directly. "I told them I saw you holding hands but Brandon, Stacey, and Bernie made up the kissing part."

"We weren't holding hands like the way you think it to be. Tom just reached out for a brief moment and held the top of my gloved hand to say thank you."

"Okay Bertha, you can go back to the unit now," she said.

"And Maria, try not to get too attached to your patients. I know you have a soft and sensitive heart but this unit is tough for anyone. You have to toughen up for your sake. I have to admit, I can't do the job you guys are doing."

At least she's honest, Maria thought to herself.

"Can I go now? Am I still in trouble?"

"Yes, you can go now and no, you're not in trouble. Maureen's husband spoke highly of you. They wrote me a glowing letter of appreciation for the work you did taking care of Maureen.

Maria went to the unit to find Holly intubated. After the lung biopsy, the doctors could not wean her off the ventilator. Her lungs were so bad the 100% Hi-flow mask was not enough to oxygenate her. Bernie was out so she had her again for the evening. In as much as she hated to see her sustained by mechanical means, at least Holly's no longer struggling to breathe. The machine was set to a certain setting to deliver artificial breaths per minute and supply her with the amount of oxygen she needed to keep her cloak of flesh alive. Unlike before when she was fighting the vent the first time she was intubated, this time, she's totally surrendered to the machine. She had given up the fight.

Maria wondered if she knew deep down that her husband was dead. Yesterday when she woke up from her morphine nap, she told Maria,

"I had a beautiful dream. I was home in Maine, sitting on the rocks by the sea looking out to the most beautiful sun before it sets below the waters. Then I woke up and saw my husband here in this room with me. I guess I was dreaming within a dream."

As she watched her breathing in synch with the ventilator, Maria felt relieved for her. She's no longer breathing through the constricted airways. With the Morphine drip, she's comfortable in the continuous infusion of opiate heaven. Listening to the rhythmic hissing sound of the apparatus, Maria can't help but wonder how bizarre life is; how boundaries between dimensions and lines of realities are blurred; how the conscious and the unconscious, the waking state and dream world all jammed up in one quantum soup. Which one is more real? She asked herself. In our waking moment are we just consciously dreaming a physical world that's as transient as the seasons, therefore not real? Maya. The Sanskrit word for illusions, a world of dreams and a false reality. We are all just living graciously with ungracious personalities in a world of dreams and when you work with folks like the gangsters of the BMT unit, the dream turns into a nightmare.

"Hey, Maria Tom called and is asking for you." Marybeth came to where she stationed herself right outside Holly's room.

"Can you tell him I'm busy. I have to go in and suction her ET tube."

"He called three times already. He knows you're on this evening."

"Okay, tell him I'll come by in a little bit."

Brandon and Stacey were at the nurse's station right across Tom's room and were giving her the most vicious looks. They were spoken to by the Nurse Manager right after Maria's meeting.

"Hey Tom, 'just came to say hi. I'm glad to see the urine is clearing up." She said standing right outside the glass wall.

"Hey stranger, where have you been?" he asked with a soft and gentle voice. "Are you avoiding me?"

"No, I was off for a week." She lied. "I'm taking care of the patient in the last room."

In the corner of her eyes, she saw Brandon and Stacey huddled in front of the computer whispering something she didn't care to hear.

One of Tom's IV pumps beeped and Brandon came, rudely brushed her aside to go in without even saying anything.

"Okay, Tom, gotta go back to my post. Get some rest." Maria said hurriedly.

The four schemers scheming to get her fired, sensed a deeper spiritual connection between Tom and Maria. But they turned something beautiful and innocent into a sordid, sleazy affair. Born of ignorance and fear of something they didn't comprehend, they created a projection of their own sordidness. In their self-righteousness, they felt superior enough to leave Maria disgraced and dishonored. They were jealous of something they don't have.

She remembered a line in T.H. White's book, 'When your honor trampled in the sewer of baser minds, learn why their tongue wags and what wags it.' Maria felt humiliated and asked herself, why do these fuckers wag their tongues? What do they eat to make them so vile, a 3-decker sauerkraut/toadstool sandwich? She's so angry but she refused to go down to their level. She tried to justify their motivation. Maybe they're intimidated by the purity of the soul connection between Tom and Maria. Maybe they're frightened, not of these two divine lovers but of who they are—meanspirited and base. They don't understand the heights and depths of the strength and courage these two ancient souls have. Their fears came from the barrenness of their hearts, their incapacity to experience the deepest low and the highest highs of human emotions.

Scorned by her colleagues, Maria found a new strength to face her nightmare. Their malevolence ignited her inner core, strengthened her resolve to remain steadfast in who she was becoming—strong in the face of any storm. Inner strength not outer armoring, she told herself. But the burden of pretense was weighing heavy on her as their proof of plasticity was more apparent. She maintained a civil façade around them but wouldn't betray herself now by cowering to these vicious pack of wolves.

Maria was completely lost in her thoughts when the alarm from Holly's cardiac monitor blasted. Her heart rhythm took a sudden turn form regular tachycardia to Ventricular tachycardia, then flat lined. She rushed into the room, pushed the code blue button and started pressing on her chest. Laura and Marybeth came with the code cart as the code team rushed in. The room was suddenly swarmed with a mix of hospital staff pumped up with nervous energy. The Nursing supervisor yelling crowd control.

"Non essentials leave the room, now!"

Laura mixed up the dopamine bag from the code cart, threaded the line and programmed the dosage into the IV pump. Marybeth quickly set up the arterial line, handed it to the resident desperately feeling for a pulse in Holly's wrist. But she's clinically dead, with no heartbeat to sustain a blood pressure, nor a pulse to be felt where the resident can insert the A-line needle through. The code nurse took over Maria, now exhausted at pumping Holly's chest without much success.

"Charge the defibrillator to 200 joules." The doctor barked at the Stat nurse in charge of the machine.

"Charging, charging. Clear!" and she placed the two paddles in her chest to no avail.

The code went on for over an hour and there was an adrenaline rush pumping through everyone's veins. It was an organized madness, the staff seemingly enjoying a high-flying sensation of having to face a medical nightmare head on. That's what seasoned nurses like Marybeth thrived on. She's stoic under pressure.

After three shocks from the defibrillator, four doses of epinephrine, a sprinkle of Atropine here and a dose of Vasopressin there, the flatline on the monitor started to quiver, throwing spikes of electrical currents forming atrial and ventricular contractions. Holly's heart was chemically revived. After having been jumpstarted, her cardiac muscles came back with a vengeance. From asystole, now its beating much faster- 260-300 a minute- with erratic beats. The cardiac monitor blaring tachyarrhythmias.

"Start an Amiodarone drip." The resident ordered.

The code team dispersed, and now gone, Maria was left cleaning up the mess. She looked at Holly suspended in lines, wires, and machines, but she's not there. Her physical body may be sustained artificially by chemical and mechanical means, but there's nothing there but a corporeal coil. Her spirit was now at home in Maine with her husband watching a golden sun setting across the Atlantic Ocean.

Maria gave report to Flambam 50 minutes past 11:00 pm. She better not complain about anything, she thought. What a nightmare the shift had been. It started with a nagging fear of getting fired and losing her job. It ended with a stark reality that life is so fragile and uncertain.

Chapter Seven

Unraveling the Lies

Maria came back the next day and met Holly's parents for the first time. The father was a respectable-looking man in his 60's, his shoulders hunched carrying a heavy weight of grief. The mother, in her fifties, was beautiful in her natural unvarnished looks. Her sad eyes looking at Holly with unshed tears, trying to hold them with the hope that she just might wake up again as she did the first time. They were the epitome of uncomplicated Northern folks living in the simplicity of provincial life, their pure hearts untarnished by the intricacies of city living.

Maria was getting report from Bernie when she saw the attending, the fellow, the resident and the intern all in pecking order came up to the parents right outside Holly's room. They were all impeccably garbed in white lab coats that denotes purity of the profession, but there's no purity in what they're selling. The desecration of the human body from radiation and chemotherapy is the ultimate antithesis of the sanctity of life. There's nothing sacred about it. Suffering in all ways and form is not what God has intended for His children. Why do humans experience it, is one existential question Maria was trying to understand.

The attending stood in the midst of the pack, his face stone cold like a freshly cut marble from the Carrara mountains, barren of any emotion as if not a ray of sunlight has shone to warm his heart. His lean stature framed in a seemingly holographic structure, like a solid ghost, yet not solid enough to feel his essence. He has a brilliant mind but his heart dull, devoid of any drop of compassion.

Bernie finished her report. "There's nothing much to tell except, oh by the way, she's still a full code."

"What?" Maria gasped. "How many more times can you beat a dead horse?"

She just shrugged her shoulders and bid Maria, "Good luck." As she took off.

The BMT team had left and the elderly couple still hovered outside the plastic wall that divided the inside from the outside. Maria got two folding chairs and brought it in for them to sit.

"Aren't we suppose to scrub in?" the mother asked nervously unsure if Maria was doing the right thing.

She was tempted to say, 'fuck the protocols, Holly can't be harmed anymore by any threat of infection.'

But she just said, "it's okay ma'am, Holly's fully engrafted. Her immune system is fully functioning."

"When do you think she'll wake up?" The mother asked Maria as she set the chairs by the window. "When will she get off of the respirator?"

She asked questions hoping against hope that she'll be answered with miracles. Like Demeter, mother of Persephone who was abducted by Hades and brought to the shadowlands, she would not grieve and move on. She's refusing to give up as her daughter lay wasted by modern medicine.

"I don't know dear, she's pretty sick. Her kidneys are failing and her liver enlarged. Her lungs are bad and she can't breathe on her own." She added, "I can't fix her lungs, I can't fix her liver, I can't fix her kidneys. I can only make her comfortable."

And the mother finally broke down in tears. Maria was filled with compassion as she hugged Holly's mom.

"What did the doctors tell you about the result of her lung biopsy?"

"They said her lungs are stiff from the GVH." The father said. "But there's a chance she might live if she gets a new pair of lungs. They suggest a lung transplant. They said to hang on as her transplant was successful."

Congratulations! The bone marrow transplant was a success, but unfortunately the patient died, was basically what the message was from the team.

'They lie!' Maria wanted to scream and tell them the doctors were giving them false hopes. But she zipped her mouth. Deep inside her was a rage. She wanted to tell them, 'They are a bunch of liars with god complex utterly lacking even a drop of respect for the sanctity of human life.'

Maria was appalled. How far would these doctors push their inhumane agenda. They are unbelievably dense in their own medical delusions. They developed protocols that aggrandized their ego, sell it out as treatments wrapped up in false hopes. Delusions of medical breakthrough box-wrapped in satin gold Pandora's box, brimming with adverse side effects and horrifying assault to the human body. There's no reverence for the sacredness of human life. What happened to the Hippocratic oath, 'First, do no harm.'

Holly's been harmed the first week of her conditioning, retching her guts out after the triple combination of chemo. On her second week her mouth and esophagus started sloughing off. She was vomiting curdled blood with dead tissue the size of a small mouse. Her upper airway was getting blocked that she needed intubation. She was on death's door maintained by a machine, sustained by chemicals. She didn't die yet, but medical technology afforded her a death rehearsal. It wasn't her time yet. She got off the ventilator as her mucous membrane healed. But this time, it's real, there's no coming off it. The sweet gentle Holly has ridden off into the sunset with her husband.

The rest of the shift seemed anti-climactic to the previous evening. Maria went about her tasks like a robot. There's nothing to engage in emotionally except her own revulsion to how doctors deal with these innocent couple. She managed to hold her inner turmoil as the parents remained in the room hoping, waiting for their daughter to wake up. But Holly was locked in, strapped in wires and machines that beeped when parameters were breached. Troubleshooting the alarms, documenting data from the monitors, maintaining drips to sustain her corporeal flesh, was not what Maria considers nursing at its essence. It's all mechanical tasks that don't require much of a heart.

Now the care has to shift to the living. Maria went to the report room and got them a mug of coffee. 'This is gonna be a long vigil,' she thought. She felt an ache seeing Holly's parents burdened with sadness and confusion. They needed to be told the real picture. Maria wanted to be honest with them but her honesty might be construed as interfering. She didn't have the courage anyways. All she can do was to pray for them to be comforted in their grief and be guided to do what's best for Holly. She was immersed in their anguish when she heard a voice, "Don't carry their grief, Maria. You weren't born to be a grief bearer. Even your own you have to release."

She drove home that night after the shift feeling washed out, drained, disillusioned. Slowly, layers of illusions were peeled off her eyes. She's questioning her own values, her motivation to work in this type of setting. She chose BMT nursing for the challenge of the complex care of cancer patients; a combination of oncology nursing and intensive care for patients undergoing hematologic procedure; either bone marrow or stem cell infusion after an intensive conditioning. She wanted to serve the best way she can in her subdued manner.

The patients coming through that double doors of the BMT unit were special in their own way. They were full of hope and courage to beat the odds, and to circumnavigate a death sentence. Maria wanted to offer support in her small way. Now she's wondering if she's an agent of death herself, administering lethal doses of toxic drugs to the patients.

She was off for two weeks and was glad for the respite from the emotional and psychological strain her work had on her. The stresses were layered coming from different sources, not just from the work itself but from dealing with toxic co-workers. They were not mean people but maybe it's their own way to vent out the pressure from a challenging work environment. Lateral violence, someone called it.

Nurses are like sponges. They absorb the stress coming from all directions not only from the patients and relatives but from doctors and colleagues. They can't lash out their frustrations towards their patients or doctors so they do it to each other in some ways.

Maria spent most of her time at the arboretum, her wooded sanctuary. Longer nights of Winter gone, the days stretched with warmer temps that brought life to stir beneath the thawing ground. In April, frequent rains softened the soil and out of a deep sleep... tulips, daffodils and crocuses shoot out of the frozen earth with ease. She's nourished by the budding greens that sprouted out of the sleeping branches. From out of the barren Winter, life surged in quiet abandon. The magnolias were garbed in thick pink velvet, the cherry blossoms burst out in profusion of white and lavender lace as if to quench her thirst; a deep thirst for something good, something real and true. Not the lies ensconced in her work that's slowly unraveled before her eyes. She remembered a line from a book, 'If you believe the lies, you won't see the truth.' For all the time she worked there, she believed the 'lies', even the one she tells herself that working there added meaning to her life. Now she could see through the lies and she didn't like it.

She walked farther towards the lilac hill. The flowers weren't out yet, but she can almost smell the heady scent of lilacs. She sensed an onrush of something from within; gentle as the morning breeze, soft as the westerly wind but felt foreboding. No matter what unfolds in her personal and work life, she'll be fine. Nature taught her to trust in a Higher Power.

She came back to work rested and ready for whatever shows up in her radar. She learned the day after she took care of Holly, the parents decided to take her off the ventilator. Few minutes later she passed away. She was expecting that but the one she wasn't ready for was the fact that Tom was now on the ventilator. She almost lost it but fought the urge to pass out.

"How did it happen?" she asked Laura. "I thought he was getting better, his counts are coming up. He stopped bleeding and was off the bladder irrigation when I left."

"He developed respiratory acidosis that he needed to be intubated, you'll know more when you get report," she said. "He's been asking about you before he was tubed," Laura added.

"Oh no, I can't take care of him," Maria insisted. "Give me the new admission in room 16."

"Are you sure? You're better off with Tom, he's in the machine. This new patient, he's a live wire."

Maria realized Laura was right. Two words summed up her shift that evening - controlled chaos. She walked into a 'rapid response' situation where the patient's heart rate fluctuated between 160-180, the heart monitor screaming SVT (supraventricular tachycardia). His blood pressure plunged down in the 80's systolic, unsustainable for a functioning heart and brain. The doctors barking orders for fluid resuscitation. His BP stabilized after 4 liters of lactated ringer, but his heart remained in the 120-130 range.

The patient was getting more agitated, screaming to his wife, "let me die now! I don't wanna do this anymore."

"Can you calm him down? And give him some pain medicine? I can't bear to see him like this." She was shaking and flailing out of her wits, too.

"So, kill me now!" the husband kept yelling. "I had enough of this. Let me go!"

The wife replied, "I love you so much. I can't let you go, not yet."

The wife was getting more distraught as the husband's escalating and becoming more combative. Maria has two patients in her hands now. She was fixing the wires on his chest connected to the cardiac monitor when all of a sudden, he sat up in the bed and grabbed Maria's arm with a vice grip, twisted it and looked straight in her eyes and vehemently yelled,

"Kill me now, or I'll kill you!"

Maria learned from past experience you can't argue with a confused patient. She found the courage to look him in the eye with all the strength she could muster and with strong authority said,

"You're hurting me. Let my arm go, NOW!"

The patient heard the power behind her words. He then released her hands and settled back in bed. What transpired at that moment was a quantum entanglement between a deranged mind and a threatened ego. How much more of this can she continue to take, she asked herself. She kept her cool as she explained to the wife.

"I've already given him a dose of Dilaudid and some Ativan," she explained. "More doses would lower his blood pressure even more."

Maria was getting tired of chasing the alarms blaring constantly, in addition to calming both husband and wife. But she has to calm herself first. She was caught in a whirlwind of chaos. Unless she controls herself, she'll fall apart at the seams and won't be able to deal with the situation. She remembered the Hermetic law of correspondence - as within, so without. The outer reality is a reflection of the inner world. True enough, after a minute of her own conscious deep breathing, she shifted her internal world from chaos to calm, and she projected a quiet energy to the wife, who dropped herself down at the recliner. Well, maybe that, or just simply from exhaustion. The husband, though, needed something else.

She asked Mindy hovering outside the room, "Hey can you ask the doctor to order vitamin H? One for him and some for her?" referring to the wife in jest.

Mindy came back with a vial of Haldol.

"How much did he order?" Maria asked

"1.25 mg." she grinned with a smirk in her face.

"Are you kidding me?"

"Just let your fingers slide." She said as she handed her the vial.

"I can't. His BUN and creatinine are through the roof."

"Well then, you just have to put up with his agitation all night. Or intubate him for bad behavior, as Brandon would say."

After a while that seemed like eternity, the combination of Dilaudid, Ativan and Haldol, the patient settled down. The wife went out to get a cup of coffee.

Maria saw the charge nurse at the report room, "Hey Laura, where's Stacey? I haven't got report from her yet."

"Her bag is gone. She looked frazzled, she must have left already." She said, "I'll give you a blur."

Maria learned that Mr. John Braveheart was a 55-years old contractor from Sommerville. He was here twice already for two mini-transplants that failed. With all the chemo and radiation, he developed a secondary cancer. Now he has AML. A modern-day Sisyphus, he's here for a third transplant but his renal function tests showed a looming kidney failure from high levels of Tacrolimus in his system. Therapeutic levels range from 5-15ng/ml but he came in with 25. His creatinine and BUN (blood, urea, nitrogen), lab tests that determine kidney function, were way above the normal values.

Tacrolimus is an inhibitor that suppresses the recipient's immune system to prevent rejection of the donor's marrow or stem cells. It's a potent anti-rejection drug however, this immunosuppression has a dark side to it. The drug causes a slew of side effects ranging from minor to major symptoms. Minor side effects include headaches, diarrhea, dysarthria, rashes, visual changes, seizures, Psychosis and behavioral changes. It increases the risk for infection and risk for skin cancer and lymphoma. One adverse effect is kidney injury.

Kidney damage is characterized by elevated waste products reflected in rising levels of creatinine and BUN. This is due to reduced GFR (glomerular filtration rate)- the body's ability to filter out unwanted elements from the body. Toxic levels of Tacrolimus cause vasoconstriction on the renal tubules leading to reduced blood flow to the kidneys. This drug-induced narrowing of the blood vessels, in turn, deprives the organ of Oxygen supply leading to ischemia which is the main mechanism in the pathological changes in kidney failure. Certain foods like oranges, grapefruit, bananas taken in excess are contraindicated to Tacrolimus. It raises the blood level of the drug in the body. And from what the wife had said, Mr. Braveheart loves grapefruit and drinks a lot of orange juice.

The lull from the Haldol and Ativan was short lived. John started waking up and the alarm from his cardiac monitor was merciless showing atrial fibrillation, his heart rate between 130-140. He wasn't as agitated, though as much as earlier. Maria paged the house officer for a different betablocker other than Metoprolol and Diltiazem, which he already had earlier but didn't seem to control his heart rate.

"Would you consider Amiodarone?" Maria suggested.

"No, just give him another dose of Metoprolol."

"By the way, he hasn't peed yet after all those IV bolus."

"Okay, place a foley catheter, see if you can get something. His kidneys are shutting down. His creatinine doubled up in 4-hour and tripling as we speak."

Maria hated inserting foley catheters especially in male patients. Although she can't confuse which hole to slide the tube through, the male anatomy has a longer corridor before the tip can reach the bladder. Where's Marybeth when I need her, she thought. She saw her friend passing by room 16 on the way to her patient.

"Mindy, can you help me insert a catheter on John? I need your emotional support."

"Sure, I'll get the supplies. Make sure to pre-medicate him. Put him in a coma first unless you want to get jumped again."

After explaining to the wife what she's about to do, Maria waited till John reached the top steps to Haldol heaven before she and Mindy went into the room. With the top of the foley lubed up with good amount of Urojet, the latex tube went in smoothly but no urine came out.

"Are you in?" Mindy asked.

"Yeah, where else can it go?"

After a long while, three drops of dark concentrated brown fluid came out.

"Jackpot. Marybeth calls it bladder sweat." Mindy chuckled.

"Thanks Mindy. Let me know what I can help you with."

"Oh yeah, I need someone to double check chemo with me. I'll meet you in room 21, when you're ready."

The new patient in room 21 was a nice doctor from New Hampshire. He was in his mid-fifties, happily married with 2 children.

After double checking the math and matching it with the protocol order, cross checking it with the dosage in the chemo bottle, Mindy and Maria went to room 21.

"Hello sir, can you tell us your full name and your birthday?" Mindy asked the patient. "We're going to hang your first dose of Cytoxan."

He also gave the two nurses his hospital ID number, memorized by heart.

"Is that your bank account number?" Maria joked.

"No, but even if I give you my bank account, you can't get enough from them. I'm just a poor doctor from New Hampshire, unlike your doctors here in Boston."

They all laughed, as Mindy programmed the infusion rate into the Imed pump located right outside the plastic wall. Maria connected the secondary tubing to the main line and spiked the chemo bottle with it, noticing the orange tag at the bottom of the bottle. It's an octagonal shaped hazard label with a skull above the X mark that says, 'Caution: toxic poison, causes cancer'. Maria's been hanging chemo and seeing that label many times before but this was the first time it hit her like a brick.

Later as the two nurses settled on their break Maria asked Mindy.

"What are we doing here Mindy?"

"Eating supper and enjoying the quiet before hell break loose again."

"No, I meant what are we doing to these patients? Doesn't it bother you when you see the caution sticker on the chemo? We are administering toxic chemicals that actually causes cancer as a side effect."

"Yeah, it does. But it's not like they were forced to receive it. Just like the doctor who's now a patient himself, they came in with full consent. Informed consent as it is."

"So, we're like James Bond? Licensed to kill. Toom, toom, doom, doom, Tadada!" Maria humming the theme song sarcastically.

"Cut it off. Sarcasm doesn't suit you."

"And oh, what about that Gelkam they put on their teeth with the nightly routine mouth care? Supposedly to prevent cavities. You know how much fluoride is in it?"

"I know." Mindy is starting to see her point. "And Fluoride is a known rat poison."

"And it calcifies the pineal gland, dumb us down if not kill us right away."

"I wonder how much does the hospital charges for a rat poison?" Maria referring to Gelkam.

"Now, don't get me started on a guilt trip. I know, the things we follow as protocols sometimes, are ridiculous. Remember when we first started here. We ask patients to do a douche every Monday and a vaginal suppository supposedly to prevent fungal infection."

"Oh yes! And your patient almost choked when she swallowed that elongated, quarter-sized suppository instead of inserting it in her vagina."

"How about your patient putting the tongue drops into her eyes, good thing she didn't get blind. And they aren't even confused."

"No, just chemo brained and irradiated."

"We've been through a lot ever since we started here."

"Remember that night when your patient came out of his room after he cut his Hickman?"

"How can I forget, he was trailing blood into the next room. Good thing he didn't wake up the patient there."

"And the resident didn't know how to sew it back together. He was reading the instructions step by step from the manual you were holding for him."

"What about the Russian paratrooper, flown for transplant from the Chernobyl meltdown. He was screaming his head off after a week of chemo and radiation."

"Poor chap. He doesn't speak English and nobody understood him. He kept yelling 'yebat!' His flying above the nuclear disaster was probably a walk in the park compared to his experience here."

"Did he ever go home?" Mindy asked.

"No, he died. A week before he died, I took him down to the ground floor for a CAT scan. He was intubated. The respiratory therapist was bagging his ET tube all the way down to the bowels of the hospital. I was 3-month pregnant pushing the heavy bed and rolling the IV poll with three pumps, the aid on the other side."

"Why didn't you put him on the stretcher?"

"Are you kidding? The stretcher's not big enough to hold the portable monitors and oxygen cylinder. And he swelled up. I was afraid he was gonna code in the elevator."

"That must have been a nightmare."

Their break ended abruptly by the alarm coming from room 16. His heart rate was up through the roof again- 170 to 180/minute, though he's sedated now. His finger oximeter showed his oxygen dropping to a dangerous level, 80-84% as his lungs were filling up with fluids from all the IV boluses he got. With his kidneys not working, he's not clearing the narcotics, no longer agitated but slipping into a semi-comatose state.

"Crap! This guy's gonna code again!" Maria squelched the fear rising up in her. "Mindy, can you page the house officer Stat. and the respiratory therapist.

Finally, the resident ordered an Amiodarone bolus, followed by a continuous drip. Maria wanted to say, 'I told you so!', but didn't.

She could have been rich by now if she gets a thousand bucks every time, she'd say that phrase.

After talking with the attending, the team decided to call the Renal Fellow to insert an access for CVVHD (Continuous veno-venous hemo-dialysis). His blood pressure was too low to tolerate a regular dialysis. To squeeze his kidneys, he ordered 60 mgs. of Lasix then a 100 mgs, when no urine came out. He followed the order with a continuous infusion of 2 mg/hour to start. The respiratory therapist put him on 50% Hi-flow. His saturation went up to 91%.

The Amiodarone drip has to be titrated down to adjust for the falling blood pressure. Dopamine was ordered to prevent it from plunging down further. Maria found herself in a high-wire balancing act between chemicals. Administer this drug to offset the side effect of the other. Do this to counter balance the other. It's a slow code, without much commotion but still kept Maria and her nursing shoes running in different directions.

Maria looked at the clock and told it to hurry. 10:45 pm. She only needs 15 more minutes before her shift ends. She's dreading the time when Dr. Gordon, the Renal Fellow who's on tonight would come to insert the CVVH catheter. She calls him Dr. G, short for god with small g. But he swaggers with a big E, his ego bigger than God. He yelled at her before for something she can't even remember now but the way she treated her, still stuck around. What are the odds that he would come at the change of shift, she wondered.

Then she saw the groundhog strolling in without its shadow. Her replacement was early. She's never been so excited to see Flambam, like the advent of an early Spring on the heels of a long Winter. Maria was relieved of the burden of dread lifted from her shoulders.

Flambam took report early. She seemed nicer than usual, accommodating almost. She sensed in her a change of heart and all of a sudden, the animosity between them was gone.

Chapter Eight

EPIPHANY

She drove home that night with a heavy sinking heart. She was so busy she didn't have time to process the shock of Tom being on the ventilator. The two weeks she was off she felt his presence but slipping away as she was walking alone at the arboretum. She reveled in the silent eloquence of the budding greens, the loud colors of azaleas screaming pink and the whisper of the Westerly wind. She rejoiced at the landscape turning from the dull grey of Winter into the vibrant ambiance of chartreuse green. However, something was amiss.

The next day she came to work, she could no longer refuse to take care of Tom. Brandon's working a short shift so Maria was assigned to him. She learned that he developed interstitial pneumonia and worsening respiratory acidosis.

"How long has he been intubated?" Maria asked.

"About two weeks now." He answered.

Maria now realized why while on vacation, she felt a tug of dread in her heart, an uneasy feeling that something was wrong.

She went into his room right after report. His wife was there sitting by his bed holding his hand. All these times that Tom was in the unit, she has never met her till now. She's very attractive, glossed up like the kind you see in Vogue covers.

"Hi. Are you Maria? Finally, I've met you. He's been talking about you a lot." She tried to shake her gloved hands. "I'm Cory, Tom's wife."

"Yes. I'm taking care of him this evening. Nice to meet you."

When Tom heard Maria's voice, he opened his eyes and a drop of tear flowed sideways. He tried to mouth some words around the ET tube and started coughing. The corrugated plastic tube that connected him to the vent was filled halfway with frothy reddish secretions.

"It's okay Tom. I'm here. Maria's here." Her voice shaking as she saw the blood coming out of his lungs.

"If you don't mind stepping out for a moment while I suction him." She said politely to the wife.

"Tom, I know you hate narcotics but I have to give you an extra dose from the Morphine drip. I Have to clear your airway and this will lower the pressure building up on the vent." The alarm from the machine was loud and disturbing adding to the emotional chaos Maria was experiencing.

He blinked his eyes as if to say yes. Maria has to stay stoic in the face of her emotional turmoil. How do you stay calm? How do you carry on with your duties when you're falling apart? But a small voice in her says, "stay centered, you're strong!"

Cory didn't come back into the room after she had seen that much blood came out of him. She went back to the hotel where she was staying while in Boston. With the extra bolus of Morphine, Tom settled in a peaceful sleep as if content that Maria was there with him. His vital signs were stable and he's breathing in sync with the vent.

Maria put on his favorite song, not too loud, not too soft, but enough to drown the rhythmic hissing of the respirator he's hooked to. She reminisced the times they spent together, the conversation they shared and how he quoted Nietzsche as if it was his own, "From which stars have we fallen to meet each other here."

The shift seemed to drag on until she saw Mindy.

"Maria, I'm ready to get report when you are."

"I was looking for you when I came in. I thought you'd be here."

"I'm here now, working the third shift."

"I'll be rotating on the night shift, too, the next schedule."

"Great. We'll both be digging in the graveyard shift." She chuckled. How are you? How is he?"

"He's stable for now and still a full code."

"I thought he made himself a DNR when he first came in. You said he didn't want to be tubed."

"Yeah. but apparently the wife persuaded him to reverse it."

"And he didn't want to do the transplant to begin with either, but she forced him into it."

Maria thought if he didn't consent to the transplant, he wouldn't be this sick. But their paths wouldn't have collided, either. For a short time, his soul had walked upon her path. She drove from work devastated, she didn't know how she got home. She felt someone's hands were in the steering wheel.

The next day she came to work, Brandon was there. She thought, great I don't have to take care of Tom. She thought wrong. Brandon was only working 7-3 again. She tried to complain about her assignment.

"Laura, can I have a different patient? Why is Brandon working the short shifts?"

"What's all these complaining about? Do as you're told, and suck it up." She was curt and dismissive.

Maria wondered if she got out of the wrong side of the bed when she woke up this morning. She's usually even keel. She learned later, her dog died.

Brandon didn't have much to say for report. Tom's wife made him a DNR and actually wants him unplugged from the machine.

Maria took it calmly. Her plan was to extubate him and let the remaining light in him burn out like a candlewick running out of wax.

"The doctor ordered Ativan and Nembutal before taking him off the vent." He said matter of fact, without any emotion.

"Where's the wife now?" Maria asked.

"She went back to the hotel with the rest of the family."

Maria nodded without a word. It will be just her and Tom alone at the final moment of his life.

Brandon left and she thought he went home but he came back with 3 bristojects; one Ativan and two 100 mg. of Nembutal. He started pushing the Ativan through the main line.

"Brandon, what are you doing? That much Nembutal will kill him prematurely." Maria was getting upset.

"Turn off the vent and disconnect him from the machine," he ordered Maria. "I'll take care of this," he added.

"Your shift is done. This is my time," she argued. "I'll do what's best for him and let nature take its own course."

Tom was still connected to the heart monitor showing a slowing heart rate-50-40-30/minute. The respirator turned off, his chest still heaving to breathe but in agonal rhythm. Then suddenly, his heart flatlined and his breathing ceased, his body engulfed in the great silence. Just like that, he was gone.

"I'll help you with the post-mortem care."

"Go home. You've done enough."

She slowly disconnected him from the monitor wires, cleared his Hickman line from the IV tubing, removed the foley catheter, as she disconnected herself from the unreality of this moment. She remembered Maureen's saying, "her body is her cross she's carrying."

Maureen carried her cross alive, home to her family but Tom was crucified in his, carrying it to heaven. She looked at his lifeless form, his pallid skin as white as the freshly fallen snow, and realized at the basic level, the physical body is no different than a claypot. It's nothing but an earthenware of desires, of longings and broken dreams. When the light that animates the vessel is snuffed out, the mortal flesh merges with the earth but where do those desires and longings go? She wondered.

Laura came in with the body bag and helped her wash him for the ritual of post mortem. She cleared the IV pumps, taking off the lines and tubing. She noticed the Morphine line was already out of the pump with the bag empty.

"Maria what happened to the Morphine bag? It's bone dry."

"Oh, I don't know. There was still a fifth in the bag when I came in at 3. And I haven't taken the line out yet from the pump. How did that happen?"

"We have to make an incident report and how do we account for the remaining morphine?" Maria asked.

"We'll just have to sign it off as wasted." She replied. "Are you okay to take him down to the morgue?"

"Yeah, I'm fine." She lied.

Maria went home distressed, confused as to whether she played the role of nurse Kevorkian. Did she kill Tom? That Morphine bag did not just empty itself and she's sure she did not touch it. Did it hasten his death? Did Brandon have something to do with it? She was so angry with herself for not being able to stand her ground? She should have been more aggressive with him and should have never let him override her decision to let Tom go naturally in his own time.

With so much guilt and anguish she couldn't sleep, sobbing so hard her chest tightening in a vise grip. She was drowning in her emotional storm, crying out,

"Oh my God, I killed him."

Nothing could ease her turmoil, even prayers seem futile. Then she remembered a shamanic meditation she often used to escape her marriage even for an hour. She listened to the rhythmic beat of the drum that put her in a trance. The voice helped her to relax and guided her through a shaman's journey. She was asked to imagine walking across a green meadow. At the far end she stopped in front of an oak tree with an opening at the base big enough for her to slide in. It was dark inside but she could see a flight of steps inside the trunk of the massive tree. The voice told her to climb up and when she reached the top, it opened up to a pristine sandy beach with a crystalline waterfall on the other side. The voice then asked her to walk towards the waterfalls where she will meet her guide.

"Do you see him now?" asked the voice.

"Yes!" Maria replied as she saw a silhouette of a luminous being so bright she can't make out the face.

"Tell me his name."

Without hesitation she replied, "Jesus Christ!"

As soon as she uttered His name, she was engulfed in the most brilliant light radiating from the resplendent Being two yards away from her. She found herself floating in the warm crystal-clear pool below the waterfall. She was cleansed of all anguish and pain. The warmth of the water comforted her. She was held in a loving, radiant essence of a benevolent Power. There was no judgment, no blame, no reproach; just a tender, effusive outpouring of unconditional love. A comforting voice whispered,

"Don't grieve the loss of the physical body for it's not real. It is of the earth's and to earth it will merge back. What's real is the flame of spirit that was in his heart."

Then she heard Tom's voice, "You didn't kill me, Maria. It was my time to go. I love you, as I loved you across multiple lifetimes."

The psychic medium was right. They weren't meant to be together, not in this lifetime. But what Tom said – 'loving her across many lifetimes', gave her a moment of truth, an epiphany. Love doesn't end in physical death as the soul is immortal. The thought comforted her and she fell asleep with dried up tears on her face, her eyelids puffed out. She called in sick the next day. That gave her three days off before she starts her night shift rotation the following week.

She came to work faced with another yet challenging situation. She and Mindy were doubled up to take care of Mr. Braveheart, who's now intubated and hooked to a CVVHD machine. Continuous Veno-Venous Hemodialysis (CVVHD) is a short-term treatment for patients with kidney failures that can't tolerate regular dialysis. It's a 24/7 slow process of removing excess fluids and filtering waste products from the blood. It reduces serum creatinine and BUN levels that aren't excreted by the failing kidneys.

The machine is a pump the size of a jukebox. A filtration system is integrated in the contraption that acts as an artificial kidney outside the body. It sucks the dirty blood from the patient via the groin line and as it crosses the filter membrane by virtue of diffusion and ultrafiltration, the waste products are washed away using a dialysate solution. The cleansed blood then is returned to the patient through the second lumen of the CVVH line.

The flow parameters, ordered by the Renal doctors according to the clinical status of the patients, have different settings—

1. Blood flow rate, the speed at which blood is pumped out from the patient and runs through the circuit.
2. Dialysate flow rate, how much solution to run per hour through the dialyzer.
3. Net ultrafiltration rate, the actual net volume of fluid removed from the patient.
4. Effluent flow rate, calculated based on the dialysate rate plus the net fluid removal.

"Maria, you deal with the CVVHD, I'll take care of the vent."

Mindy's face reflected the confounding mess of jumbled wires and tubes and gadgets the patient was attached to. The ventilator was on the right side of the bed, the CVVH machine on the upper left side with the A-line set up beside it. Cardiac monitor hanged above his headboard and four IV poles flanked his bed two on each side, clustered with Imed pumps looking like a Christmas tree.

"It's a jungle in here." She said, "I don't even know where to begin."

"It's more like a crypt with high grade medical cobwebs!" Maria joked.

"First off. Assessment. Assess the mess!" Maria laughed at the absurdity of it all. "I'm just glad you're with me, Mindy!"

Braveheart was buried alive in crisscrossing wires and tubes coming from every orifice in his body; Endotracheal tube in his mouth; three-lumen intrajugular line on his left neck; Arterial line on his right wrist; Femoral line for CVVH; foley catheter in his penis; EEG wires plastered in his head; cardiac monitor wires on his chest that you have to straighten out, otherwise it gives a fuzzy tracing; lines, lines, lines that you have to trace to which IV pump it's connected to. One is for Dopamine drip, one for Levophed, and the other is for Morphine y-sited with the line for Antibiotics.

"At least he's stable with two pressors."

"Don't speak too soon. He's maxed out on Dopamine and the Levophed is getting up there, too."

Maria concentrated on the CVVHD. She looked at the current setting of parameters. The blood flow rate which was the volume of blood passing through the filter was at 100 mL/minute. The dialysate rate was at 2000 mL/hour, which gave her an hour and a half before replacing a new 3Liter bag. The system was taking out 100 mL/hour of fluid from his body.

She was about to draw blood to check his electrolytes and Ionized calcium when the patient started seizing, his whole body shaking under the weight of the wires and IV lines, his nose oozing blood, his BP dropping even lower.

"Mindy page the house officer. I'll give him Ativan for now."

The resident wearing his pajama scrubs rolled in.

"I was just about to take my beauty nap, what's up?"

"Hey, Dr. J, we're glad you're on tonight." Maria calls him Dr J. short for Jaworski and mostly for his joyful disposition.

He ordered IV Keppra and maxed out the Levophed. Leave- 'em-dead, as others call it, as it has nasty side effects. It causes severe vasoconstriction that increases the blood pressure even higher. He also ordered Vasopressin drip to sustain his BP while his bodily fluids were being pumped out.

"Where are we gonna run it through?" Mindy asked the resident. "All of his access are tied up."

"Page the IV nurse to insert a long line. Maria, ask the renal house officer to reduce the ultrafiltration rate."

"How much Calcium and Potassium can we give him?" Maria inquired. "His last K is 2.9 and his ionized calcium is 0.6"

"Give him 100 meq of IV Potassium and 2 grams of calcium IV. That's why he's seizing, his calcium is low. And draw his labs every 2 hour."

"Will you change the order for the sliding scale so we don't have to page you every two hours?" Mindy asked.

"Sure, you got it."

Maria turned down the ultrafiltration rate to 50 mL/hour and with the third pressor, his BP stabilized in the 100's systolic.

"Hey, Maria did you notice this dark grey, blackish lesion on his face earlier?" she asked as she suctioned the ET tube.

"I've seen a couple on his forehead. Why?"

"It seems like it's spreading down his neck. Come take a look."

"Oh, my God. That's septic emboli, maybe fungus."

"How do you know?"

"I've seen that kind in a patient I took care of when I was at Baylor Hospital in Dallas."

"Page the resident again. He needs an antifungal medicine."

Dr. J strolled in a bit annoyed. "What happened to not paging me every two hours. It's not even an hour yet. Can't you guys let me sleep?"

Maria waved her right arm over the inert body of Mr. Braveheart covered in fungal warts, his body entangled in wires.

"Behold the masterpiece of modern medicine! In trying to defeat death, we desecrate life."

The two nurses showed him the lesions popping like mushrooms, now on his arms and legs. He confirmed what Maria had thought. He ordered Micafungin.

"That Mica-fuckin-fungin is not compatible with Morphine or the other pressors. How do we administer it? Make him drink?" Mindy blurted out.

"Well, he's got another arm. Get the IV nurse to insert another long line on his left antecube." And he disappeared going back to his quarters.

An hour later, his blood pressure started dropping again and his heart rate up to 200/minute. More fungal lesions appeared on his trunk.

"Mindy, we're cultivating a fungus farm here. He's clearly in septic shock. He's gonna crash before the end of the shift."

Dr. J came back worried this time. He ordered an epinephrine drip.

"Keep him even Maria, don't take any more fluids right now. We have to stabilize his BP."

"We're out of IV access, the only access we have is the femoral line for the CVVH. We can't violate it without permission from the Renal fellow." Maria said gravely.

"Dr. J, you gotta call the attending and his wife. He's going down fast." Mindy chimed in. "We need an order to make him a DNR."

"Okay. I'll call the attending first and then his wife. Maria, call the Renal fellow."

It's 3:30 am. Maria dreaded the call but she had to. She knew the fellow on call was Dr. G. She just has to suck it up and brace for impact.

"Hello Dr. Gordon. I hate to call you at this hour but we need an order to use the CVVH line. He's now on three pressors and he's blood pressure continues to drop. The resident ordered an epinephrine drip but we're out of IV access except the CVVH line."

"Hello." He was gruff, and his voice garbled like he's just coming out of the grave. Then realizing what he was woken up for, yelled at Maria.

"No! and how dare you wake me up at this time when you know you can't use that catheter for anything except CVVH."

"I wouldn't want to indulge your wrath at this hour but we need his groin line to run a 4th pressor. He's a full code right now."

"Absolutely not!" he cut her off angrily.

Maria's getting revved up, "He's gonna crash and he needs that epi drip. It's ready to go, we just need a line."

"How many times can I say NO! That line is dedicated for only and only CVVH only. Are you dense?"

"How good is that line if the patient is dead." Maria's own supply of adrenaline was pumped up.

"How dare you! Who are you challenging my authority."

Finally, Maria had enough of his arrogance. All the frustrations, repressed anger and disappointments built up over the years had climaxed up to the point where she found the courage to tell him.

"Dr. G, this is just a courtesy call. I am not asking you, I am informing you out of respect that we are violating your sacred catheter!" Dickhead, she added as she slammed the phone so hard. It felt good, really good.

Mindy was grinning ear to ear. "Whoaah, where did that come from? You slammed that phone so hard, and loud you've woken up the dead."

"Yeah, I've roused him from his grave alright."

Maria laughed releasing some load off her chest. A bucket full of stress was emptied from her. The two nurses were laughing when Dr. J came to tell them that the attending changed his full code status.

"His wife is on her way in. She consented to the DNR."

"Do we still have to run the epi?"

"No. Start peeling off the pressors."

"What about the CVVHD?"

"Just keep going with the current settings till the wife gets here."

"Thank you, Dr J. for convincing the attending and the wife."

"You guys were the ones who convinced me. It would have been a mess coding him at the change of shift. Thank you."

Maria couldn't control herself and said what's in her mind.

"Did we convince you, too, that this is not an ideal way to treat these patients. There must be a better way. Maybe one day you'll find a more humane method."

"I agree. BMT is a barbaric treatment for cancer patients."

From the mouth of a doctor himself, Maria was glad she's not the only one that sees the procedure in a horrifying light.

Maria kept the machine going. She was amazed at the brains who invented the technology. It prompted her when to replace the dialysate bag, told her when the effluent bag is full and needed to be emptied, and when to change the filter tubing, which was supposed to be this morning.

"Maria, aren't you lucky. You're spared the headache of changing the whole filter set."

"Yeah. And you know what Mindy? I just had an epiphany."

"What? This better be good.""Think about it. The CVVH machine is another pump aside from the heart that circulates blood throughout his system. This second pump outside the body accelerates the circulation of fluids as well as the septic emboli, spreading it and popping the fungus all over his skin."

"That's probably why his body is covered with lesions in a short period of time."

"And how do you kill a dying man?"

"Put him on CVVHD?" Mindy said gravely.

The wife came in around 6:30 am and told them to stop everything and disconnect his husband from all the monitors and gadgets. Five minutes later, he expired. The two nurses got busy plucking tubes out of Mr. Braveheart.

"This guy would need a major post." Maria mumbled with clenched teeth disgusted at what they were doing. The image of an ashen grey bloated man covered in warts would haunt her for days. Once you see the horrors of how patients go through after transplant, you cannot unsee them.

"What post? I thought the wife said no autopsy."

"I meant post aesthetics. You know when the family hires someone to groom the dead for the wake."

"You mean a mortician?"

"Exactly. This guy needs a real pro to cover up this gruesome body." She was looking at his puffed-out face, mottled and disfigured.

With the CVVH stopped, his body swelled up even more, covered with grey lesions.

"What for? He doesn't care how he looks. He'll be six feet under."

"Mindy, you have to conform with society. You can't let people see him like that. They'll have nightmares."

"Why can't people just accept things as they are. Why's pretensions so fucking necessary? He's dead." Her voice trembled as she spoke the words with gravity.

Maria could sense she's starting to get disturbed as she was after what they have just experienced in the short shift.

"You groom the dead, Mindy, for the benefit of the living."

Ten minutes before 7 am, the morning shift started trekking in.

"Hey girls, how did your night go?" Laura asked.

"Fabulous." Maria replied with sarcasm.

"Mindy, we've done enough." Maria added. "I'm not going down to the morgue, not for the second time this week. Let the morning shift take him down."

"Me, neither."

The two friends left the unit together exhausted but relieved they averted a code.

"This calls for a celebration. I know of an Irish pub open at 8 am. Are you up for a pint?" Mindy asked.

"Sure! I don't drink but after last night, I might need a pint or two."

Chapter Nine

Liberation

Maria and Mindy went to the North End and found a Pub open 24-hour. The city was just waking up so traffic was minimal. They found street parking right in front of the Irish Pub. An Irish restaurant in the North end was unheard of in the old days, but gone are the days when Boston was caught in a cultural clash between the Irish and the Italians. They both have strong cultural identity that for a time, can't seem to co-exist in a small city. Now it's all mingled up in one heterogenous community thriving in diversity. Their influence, though, is still alive in their own corner of the city. The Southie is the Irish territory while the North end is the little Italy.

"You guys looked like you've just come out of the graveyard shift."

"Yeah, and we dug two graves." Maria replied, the second one she's referring to the renal fellow she had woken up.

The bartender stopped his chore mopping the other side of the room and welcomed them. They were the only ones in the pub. It reeked of alcohol binged from the previous day. He cleared a table by the window looking out on the streets. "Rough night, eh?" He sounded Canadian.

"Yeah, we need your strongest ale." Mindy said.

"What are we celebrating?" he asked.

"Liberation day!" Maria said, "last night was my last shift at the BMT unit."

"What?" Mindy's eyes opened up so wide, surprised. "When are you gonna tell me?" She sounded hurt.

"Yeah, I meant to tell you last night but we got so busy."

"I'm gonna miss you. What are you going to do?"

"I've joined the float pool and took a 24-hour night position." She said brimming, "and I got accepted at Northeastern University. I'll start the MSN-MBA program this Summer."

"Wow, congratulations! You're doing both Nursing and Business Administration?" she clinked her glasses to Maria's. "This really calls for a celebration."

"Thank you. Yeah, it's a dual program. I don't start till after a week. Tomorrow I'm going to a silent retreat in Barre, Mass. You wanna come?"

"No, thanks. I'll go crazy after a day without talking."

"I hope you don't mind me asking, but how are you going to pay for this program? The hospital doesn't give much for tuition reimbursement and you're getting divorced."

"They gave me a minority scholarship. I just have to maintain a high GPA."

"How's your divorce proceedings, by the way?"

"I fired my lawyer. She was planning on dragging the process. She only gave me 100. dollars out of the 5K retainer's fee I gave her."

"Crocs! Bottom feeders, they are the vilest of swamp dwellers."

"Luckily, I found an old guy. He just charged me 3K. I think I'm his last client before he goes to Florida to retire." Maria chuckled. "How about yours?"

"I didn't go through with it. I don't want my kids to suffer the consequence."

"I know. That's the hardest part. But my daughter is strong and smart. She knows what's going on even if she's not told of anything."

"You only got one kid. I got three. Besides he's good with them."

"Yeah, I met him once. He seemed like a sensible guy. My husband actually isn't too bad. He's just stunted. He drowns his emotions with alcohol."

The waiter came to check on them.

"How's everything? Can I get you anything else?"

"Food is excellent, we're good thank you. We just need the check please." She added, "Maria, I'll take this. Congratulations again, and here's a toast to a new chapter of your life. Wish you the best of luck."

Mindy has always been gracious and kind to her. She's grateful for the warmth of her friendship and her thoughtfulness. They parted with tears in their eyes.

The next day Maria went west of Boston. She's been driving over two hours but there's no sign yet to Barre. She was told the drive was about two hours from the city. She must have taken the wrong exit from the highway and found herself in the rough area of Worcester, a small metropolis in Central Massachusetts. There was a liquor store up ahead, the only business establishment amidst rundown dilapidated houses. She stopped to ask for direction. A grubby looking guy with unkempt long hair and beard, came out holding a 6-pack Budweiser on his chest. He grinned at her. Looked at her intently as if she was his next meal.

She set her fear aside and asked him anyways. "Hello, can you show me how to get to the Buddhist retreat center?"

He grinned wider, showing four teeth missing from the rest of his tarred, cigarette-stained chompers. Gargling his spit, he mumbled, "I don't know nottin of a Buddha camp here. You're way off miss."

Maria scurried back to her car, swearing never to stop at a liquor store for direction. She'll just have to go back to the main highway. After three hours of several wrong turns and driving back and forth, second guessing herself, she finally saw the sign to the Buddhist Center.

After another hour she reached her destination. The town's motto of "tranquil and alert" written in a plaque below a statue, fits perfectly the pastoral impressions of the town.

She passed the populated area of Barre and 2.2 miles north of the town center, she found the place. It's a large brick building situated in a serene setting with two large beige columns in front right before the entrance. It's a gateway to a different world and once you cross it, you leave behind the noise of where you came from. She was late for the registration which ended at 5 pm and missed the orientation and tour. The girl on the front desk gave her the map of the grounds with the layout of the buildings. She showed where her room was in the 'Catskills' dormitory and was told she was rooming in with a girl from Athens.

"When do we stop talking?" she whispered to her afraid she might be violating the silent mandate already.

"It's 6:30 pm now. In 30 minutes, we'll observe silence for the whole duration of the retreat except for the mid-week class with the teachers. But only the teachers can talk."

She handed her the schedule for the entire stay and added,

"We assign each person a specific task during the retreat. Your voluntary job is to cut vegetables and help with meal prep. After you put your things in your room go straight to the kitchen."

The small rectangular room with 2 small beds was bare but clean, like the ones you see in a cloister. There's not much space between the beds except for a chasm of silence.

She proceeded to the kitchen where the volunteers were busy chopping away the vegies for tomorrow's meal.

"I'm sorry I'm late." Maria addressed the six people in the room.

The kitchen manager just smiled and handed her an apron. He continued on and showed them how the vegies should be cut.

"We still have 15 minutes before we stop the chatter. I'll take this time to explain things." He said gently.

"Cut the celery in fine pieces like this but don't cut your finger along with it. There's no chance of a mishap if you're vibing positively and focused on what you're doing, unless your mind is elsewhere." He added, "If you do cut something other than the vegies, you have to let us know."

Maria thought, 'Oh, like I'll keep a bleeding thumb a secret. I'll be screaming in pain and breaking the bow of silence.'

"You wonder why we ask you to volunteer for a task. This is part of your Vipassana training. Meditation doesn't just happen sitting in a lotus position. It bleeds into everything you do- cooking, eating, cleaning, walking. It's being present, aware and alert in whatever you're doing."

Maria thought, talk about bleeding, how do you not bleed from the vicissitudes of life. She's been bleeding out from stress, anger, frustrations, grief for so many years at work and in her personal life. She came here to un-bleed.

"Vipassana is the practice of mindful doing by staying in the present moment, seeing things as they are without judgment or any interpretations the mind conjures." He continued.

Then a loud gong interrupted him in mid-sentence. It signaled the start of an interesting journey into the center of a noiseless world. She remembered when her patient muted herself and stayed inside her chatter-free box for days. Now she herself was on the threshold of it.

The first day, at 5:45 am, she was woken up by the sound of a bell that kept louder and louder, then fainter and fainter as the guy ringing the bell moved towards the next building to wake up the retreatants sleeping there. There were 70 total and with a limited shower stall, she hurried to take the first warm water before it ran out and changed to cold shower.

Breakfast consisted of boiled eggs, lentil soup and dry crackers. The dining room with 70 people was quiet except for the clang of the silverwares against the dishes and the dings and dongs of the pots and pans in the kitchen. Her lips were sealed to talk but her mind was loud, churning up worried thoughts running in different directions. Can she do this for seven days? She's thinking about her daughter she left with a friend. How is she doing? How could she juggle work, school, and family life?

The gong signaled the start of the first session of practice. The day was structured with alternating sitting and walking meditation; sit, walk, lunch, sit, walk, tea, sit, walk, sleep. Repeat the next day.

Her first sitting meditation was uneventful but with the sweet potato stew for lunch, she was sitting uncomfortably in her coccyx, feeling bloated and gassy. She felt a fart coming on. She tried to stifle it. Any noise, however faint, would reverberate across the silent hall. She stood up, left the hall before she could embarrass herself and started her walking meditation early.

The grounds weren't manicured but there's a sublime simplicity to it that lends to a peaceful surrounding. She headed towards the round garden with the statue of the buddha at the center. The irises were in full bloom, regal in their purple and pink petals. The daisies scattered around the statue were of different colors creating a rainbow of June flowers. They were not quiet nor bashful about their beauty. They screamed of their splendor and glory. The aspen trees on the other side of the walking trail, rustling their leaves at the touch of the North wind, welcomed her like a long-lost child. The place spoke to her of peace.

On her second day, she was more settled in the routine. But she asked herself, what's the point of all these? The answer came as a whisper; 'To learn to pay homage to the present moment, mindful of every action. Mindfulness is the act of showing up for life, not missing out on what is, not suppressing what's painful. Embedded in the practice is the intention of understanding the experience without judgment.'

Sitting in quiet stillness, the hall was wrapped in silence except for the whistling sound of the breeze blowing in through the open windows, and the flapping of the leaves from the birch trees outside. Then suddenly someone started sobbing wildly. She wailed unabashedly, letting go of all her dammed-up despair. A tear rolled down Maria's cheeks.

She felt her pain and everyone there empathizing with her, too. There's a sense of collective empathy permeating the entire space, demonstrating the Universal law of oneness. All is one and one is all. They were all there looking for ways on how to deal with their own suffering and to understand what makes them human.

Maria tried to control her thoughts and emotions but a voice inside her broke her meditative state.

"Don't repress it. Your thoughts are like clouds drifting across the sky. Let it go. You're not the clouds. You are the vast sky that holds them. You're not your feelings, either, but that's what make you human. Just experience it. Let it flow till it dissipates in its own time. Your emotions are your energy in motion. It has to move, otherwise, you'll be a stagnant pool of turbid waters. Pain, sorrow, grief are just fleeting energies that reflects your state of mind. But they are not you. Just observe them; today I feel joy, embrace it; now I feel pain, be present with it and it will pass; Sorrow visited me, let it stay for a few days but don't let it take space permanently; grief came, don't dwell on it. In your ever-changing inner landscape, there's a still point of strength, of joy, of peace. That is who you really are. Meditation is not about controlling your thoughts and feelings. It's connecting to the silent watcher within."

The voice continued on. "The challenges and difficulties you faced are just initiations. They are tests on how steadfast you are in your faith. You've passed them, but there will be other tests. You're being prepared to step up the next rung of your ladder."

The following day was cold and drizzly. Dark heavy clouds blowing in from the Catskill mountains made the place even more somber. It seemed like Winter in the middle of June except there was no snow. The chore of chopping vegies was becoming an adventure in itself. Cutting the carrots and the cauliflowers in the same size required precision and focus. She's more than focused now, she felt she could splice an atom. Mindful dicing of the eggplants became as exciting as any sports. Maria and the other six volunteers worked in silent cooperation with a spirit of goodwill. She was glad she wasn't given the task of washing dishes or cleaning the showers and toilets.

Lunch was served with stir fry vegies and tofu with chocolate pudding for dessert. In the meditation hall she sat close to the back door for easy exit. In the quietude of the room, she heard a grumbling sound coming from within, like rambling clouds in a thunderstorm in the quiet of the night.

She wondered, "is it me or the guy sitting cross-legged next to me?"

"It's yours," said the voice inside her. "Your tummy's not happy about the vegan stuff you're eating."

Then she heard another one, louder this time like a croaking frog trapped in a sewer.

"It's his." Said the voice, "his belly's not happy either."

She started laughing inaudibly, trying to squelch it. She's losing the piety of the moment. She was glad to hear the bell, ending the session and the cramps in her legs from sitting in lotus position.

The rain stopped but the grounds were still soggy for walking outside. Some walked in the hallways of the dormitory, some circled around the tables in the dining room, most remained in the meditation hall. It's weird watching them walk with heads bowed looking at every step moving forward with focused awareness. The sobbing lady, now in a better state, smiled at her and gravitated to her for the rest of the afternoon.

As she walked around, disturbing thoughts came flooding in as she looked at the dark clouds outside. She's anxious about her new job, worried how she could raise her daughter alone, doubtful of her capacity to take on grad work. Then she heard the voice again.

"Maria, your busy mind is the veil that dims the shine of your heart light. Relax into your surroundings. Too much thinking befuddles the mind. Your thoughts create ripples in your being that murk the clarity of your essence. Over analysis leads to paralysis... of what? ...of your heart muscle's ability to appreciate the world around you. Think a little, feel a lot. It is in your feeling side of life that you will be given the key to open all doors to beauty, peace, love, joy and abundance."

The following day, the sun came out with the winds blowing the grey clouds eastward. In the clear bright day, the sacredness of the place was magnified and everything was illumined to sparkle in the light; the leaves of the trees have greater shine, the grass much greener. The blue iris looked much bluer in the mid-day sun. A cardinal, shining in its red plumes, darted in and out of the lilac bush with the remaining blooms. Every leaf, every flower, every blade of grass was radiant with its lifeforce. She wondered if this heightened perception is an effect of meditation. As she walked around the garden, she noticed something in her hair. By instinct, she thought of squashing the bug, but the Buddhist precept of non-harming came to her quicker than her knee-jerk impulse. Then it migrated down to her left shoulder and flew upwards. She realized it was a white butterfly. She came back, sat on the back of her hand, then fluttered away to find a better perch. Maria had never felt so alive and open to life around her.

One of the lessons in the mid-week class was creating a space for receiving; being aware of sensations and feelings, recognizing it, accepting it with gratitude but not getting attached. The teachers helped her understand the lessons of acceptance, non-identification, non-harming, and non-attachment. They emphasized the Buddha's teachings on the source of suffering- clinging to things, people and memories of the past.

"Only when you can learn to let them go, can you create space for grace that's readily available for the taking," said the voice inside her.

Maria's getting used to sitting cross-legged for an hour. She's now more aware of her thoughts getting sparse and few in-between. By now, she's attuned to the voice that popped in and out, this time applauding her progress. She whispered.

"When you sit still and your mind is settled, free of the rippling tides of scattered thoughts, it's like the clear pond water. You can see the bottom. The space between your thoughts is not an empty void but a womb of creation, of abundance not lack, of Presence not absence. Silence is the open door to your inner dimension."

The meditation hall was particularly warm with the sun out. The back door was wide open to let the breeze in and so too for other living things, an invitation to join in. A baby snake crawled across the threshold, through the back door and slowly slithered towards the altar. Someone stood up, picked up the creepy crawler by its tail in reverence and escorted out of the room. The Buddha would be proud. His teachings on respecting all lifeforms, that all in existence is sacred, lives on. Maria wished it's practiced where she works.

Lunch was served with eggplant parmesan and linguine. The pasta was so good, she consumed more than she needed. Now she's draggy and lethargic. After her daily chore of chopping vegies, she sat outside the kitchen in the eastern part of the building where there's a patio facing a grassy incline. Five yards away is a wall of massive pine trees 3-4 story high, their foliage spread across like the wings of a jumbo jet. They lined up like a towering hedge to a fortified sanctuary, a forest set on a steep incline at the base of a mountain. She was mesmerized by the conifers as they swayed gently to the wind.

She closed her eyes enjoying the warm refined air blowing from the trees and she listened to the birds. They sounded much chirper than the first day she came. Something buzzed like a bee but it was far more splendid than a bee. She opened her eyes and saw a blue-green hummingbird hovering in front of a red trumpet vine nearby. She hasn't seen a hummingbird before, but she's been fascinated by how the shamans perceive them as a totem animal. They carry a message from the spirit realm; to sip only from the sweet nectar of life and to embrace new opportunities for growth no matter what the situation brings. She was amazed at how it flapped its wings so fast she can only see the fuzzy form. It hovered above the red flower, flew backwards and sideways. A symbol of adaptability and flexibility, the language they speak is that of love and freedom.

It flew away as the chipmunks and squirrels came out of their hiding, chasing each other, disappearing into the trees and reappearing back hungry, looking for food. One came up to her and ate nuts out of her hands. She's no Francis of Assisi but communing with these animals, gave her a sense of how he felt experiencing oneness with all lifeforms. These critters are friendly, she thought. They must be Buddhists, too.

A couple of dragonflies flew by in synchronous flight. They zigged and zagged in mid-air, skirting each other in a mating ritual. Then the blue dragonfly mounted the red one, grabbed her head, and started biting and scratching showing male aggression in high acrobatic fashion. This, to the female dragonfly is not true love but pure domination. She wanted nothing of it. She managed to get untangled and dropped on the ground remaining motionless. The blue dragonfly, thinking she's dead, floated above her, disappointed. He wasn't aware of the frog just waiting for the kill. In one sweeping motion, the toad stuck his tongue out and swiped the dragonfly into his belly. The tempest of unbridled, unrequited passion brought him to his own demise. The female dragonfly on the ground stirred and flew away. She faked her death to avoid unwanted copulation.

Maria was awestruck by the female dragonfly's ability to take control of her destiny. She relinquished the need to be chosen and found her power to choose her own experience, not from the clamor of carnal needs but from a space of self-respect. She belonged to no one but herself. Her worth was not measured by how others desire her but how deeply she can connect with the depth of her being. She's no longer trading self-love with superficial sex. She wanted a holy encounter not just a casual coitus in mid-air.

Sex and death played out in a serene setting, was the most dramatic scene Maria had witnessed at the retreat. That was the closest to sex she experienced vicariously in two years. Sitting alone on a bench at the back of the kitchen, facing the great green wall, she's a solo spectator in an open-air theater watching the natural world streaming in real time. Then she saw a guy walked across towards a small clearing in between the trees. He disappeared into the woods and unlike the chipmunks, he didn't come back out, as if swallowed by the dense forest. They were told to stay within the marked areas in the walking trail and not go up the mountain. She wondered why did he break the rule? What's up there?

The last day came. But she sensed a homecoming as if she has just arrived. The final sitting meditation seemed like a return to one's home, an experience of arriving at oneself. She found her mind less cluttered, more spacious, much clearer. She found a way to live beyond love and hate, beyond hope and fear. In the darkness of the void, she realized one does not find peace. One arrives at peace.

That night Maria's feeling weird. The energy generated during the meditation, now was about to burst. The fire in her belly needed an outlet. She scribbled these words in a napkin.

'Looking for God in the wrong places: I knocked at someone's door looking for God, but He wasn't there. I climbed up trees and mountains searching for Him, only to see a shadow. I sailed to distant shores and foreign lands hoping to find Him waiting, but only saw a glimmer of him. Anywhere and everywhere...He's nowhere! But the moment I sit still, I realized He is there beside me, behind me, in front of me and deep within.'

Throughout the seven days of intense meditation, diving deep into the sacred silence, she built up so much energy she needed to discharge the electrical buzz running up and down her spine. Instead of joining the group in the mess hall now chattering away, she walked out of the Buddhist retreat and ran the street heading South. It's the most rural part of town and you see nothing but trees and green lush vegetation. This is part of the Mohawk trail, also known as the Mohican trail, a 69-mile scenic byway that runs east to west originating from the Hudson River valleys in New York to the Connecticut river valleys in Massachusetts.

The road was deserted. There's no weekend traffic except a few rabbits and squirrels hopping alongside her. Fed by an unknown force, she ran for miles and ran some more until her legs can no longer carry her farther. She felt like Forrest Gump in the middle of route 32, now running on empty. She collapsed on the side of the empty road as her head whirled like a pinwheel. In her spinning world, multiple lifetimes converged in one singularity. Her many past lives carrying ancient wounds re-surfaced to be healed. She exhausted herself of old stories still haunting the dark alleys of her subconscious mind and right there at the middle of nowhere, she released every erg of negative energy clogging her body. It's her moment of liberation. She liberated herself from all the stress accumulated in all the years she worked at the transplant unit. The burden of grief, hatred, of pain and suffering she absorbed from other people was gone. She dropped the heavy weight that wasn't hers to carry. What's left was clarity and buoyancy.

Going back to the center, she wondered if she could take an Uber, or if there's even an Uber in Barre. It took her longer to get back, her legs now dragging. Half of the retreatants were gone. She asked the girl at the front desk about her roommate.

"What happened to my roommate? I've only seen her once."

"She went up the mountains. There's a forest refuge up there."

"Oh, that's where the guy went. I saw him disappeared behind the trees."

"If you want to come back and stay up there for three months."

"Wow. Those are serious meditators. Hard core. I could barely finish the seven days."

She drove home later that day feeling high on her own supply, as if she's flying faster and higher than her car. Like the hummingbird, there was an incredible sense of lightness in her with the baggage she's been carrying dropped off. The Buddha said, it's not what you gain in meditation that has more value but what you've lost in the process—anger, anxiety, worry, ill-will, hatred. Now she's ready to start a new chapter. Her world has been made new. Along the way she reflected on what the voice had said about having to face more tests. Was it a foreshadowing of things to come?

Chapter Ten

Annus Horribilis

"It was the best of times. It was the worst of times. It was the age of wisdom. It was the age of foolishness. It was the season of light. it was the season of darkness." Charles Dickens wrote these words in 1859 in his book- 'A Tale of Two Cities- when France was consumed by darkness brought on by the French revolution. But he could have written these lines for this era. 161 years later, a different darkness came rolling in across the lands. The pandemic came and Maria's reality and eight billion others were hijacked. The world lulled in complacency was shaken to its core. Chaos and confusion ruled as the season of fear and ignorance undermined the light of hope and wisdom. The architect of chaos, though unseen, wreaked terror in every one's mind and heart. Fear became the dominant force that has thrown people into uncertainty. Families were locked down in their homes for safety and as the streets were emptied, the once vibrant city of Boston now morphed into a ghost town. To vax or not to vax wasn't the question for it was mandated. The minority who refused to play along and went against the tide of vaccination, became the outliers in the field of conformity.

The world was churned about and turned inside out but there's an upside to the story. With prolonged lockdowns, pollution was paused. With fewer vehicles on the road, the earth breathed less fumes and the air was purified to some degree, while rivers and streams cleared up. It was the best thing that ever happened to the environment.

Maria loved driving the empty streets to work. The 30-minute commute shortened in half the time. Joining the float pool staff was exciting at first, as she worked in different units each week; taking care of different set of patients, working with different nurses. It's like sailing from one island to another embarking on different shores and working with different kind of natives. She learned to be more flexible and adaptable to the new work environment. She only worked two long shifts a week so she didn't mind floating around the unfamiliar units. The remaining days, she walked the grounds of Northeastern university, straddling two departments of higher learning—Nursing and Business Administration.

It was the best of time for her intellectually. Her mind was stretched to a higher level and she enjoyed collaborating with other grad students on academic projects. She wasn't sure if she could do it; juggling work, school and family, but she persisted to the point where she forced herself into a state of being delusional, not from a place of arrogance but of faith in a Higher Power. Her daily mantra was 'fake it till you make it.' Immersed in a whirlwind of academic work, she didn't have time for the pain of going through the divorce. She buried her face on books, a potent distraction to the reality of her marriage that's about to end.

Maria was getting used to the unpredictable work assignments. As she embraced the challenge of working in different units, she found a new strength and confidence. She sensed an invisible hand guiding her to tackle any challenging situation and steering her away from unpleasant work experience. At times she's spared from working in a busy unit that was mired in shit-hitting-the-fan type of madness. When she would arrive at a particular unit she's assigned to, at the last minute, she's pulled away to work in a different area. Or when she's supposed to admit a 'train wreck' patient from another hospital, the patient gets diverted to another facility. There's a Higher Power in control of her life that she's now starting to trust and surrender to. She believed nothing can happen, either good or bad, but for her highest good.

Balancing family, grad school and work, all is well in her world until the unexpected turn of events happened. When Covid hit, the hospital changed one of the step-down units into SPU (Special Pathogens Unit), and the float pool nurses would staff the covid unit. She found herself as she left the BMTU, jumping from the hot pan right into the fire.

She drove to work one day, enjoying the less congested curb of Jamaica way, yet dreading another shift at the Covid mine field, she arrived at the unit greeted with a pleasant surprise.

"Hello there, stranger!" Mindy exclaimed. "You never came back to visit me so I came to join you."

"Oh, wow! Mindy, I'm so glad to see you. Are you working here now? Is this your first night?"

"Yeah, you have to show me where things are. This is much bigger than the transplant unit."

"Yup, the rooms are more spacious and a lot more daunting. Welcome to the underworld."

The charge nurse looked at them disapprovingly. "Enough chitchat, go get report on your patients."

"We'll catch up later." Mindy said.

"Okay, hope we don't get slammed with admissions."

And so, the two friends were re-united again, working side by side as they did before. The covid unit was quiet that night, so the staff had a chance to reflect on the state of affairs going on in St. Johnswart hospital.

"Are you guys going to the MNA meeting next Monday?" Camille asked Mindy and Maria digging into their cobb salad.

"No, I have to prepare for a power-point presentation for my class that evening." Maria replied.

"You have to attend," Carol demanded. "We all have to go. This is our chance to show solidarity. That day we hand in the ballot to vote for a strike."

"What time?" Maria asked.

"9 am. We can all go after the shift." Camille replied.

"Yeah, it's time to show the big shots running this hellhole that we, nurses aren't pushovers." Carol deliberated on, "we've been working for two years without a contract. The administrators are stonewalling us, refusing to give us a raise, while they have their huge bonuses. How fair is that?"

There was rage in her voice, speaking like a true revolutionary. In her past life, she may have been part of the Boston tea party scheming for deliverance from the tyranny of the British.

"And the VP of Nursing, instead of siding with the nurses, she's even proposing to dissolve the MNA." Camille added.

"They cannot just get rid of the MNA. The organization has its own clout and influence. Unlike other hospitals in Boston that don't have labor union, this facility would not allow it." Mindy finally spoke up.

"By the way," Camille interjected, "have you heard of stories from nurses about a suspicious guy wearing a black hoodie following them to either harass or bribe them to vote no on strike."

"Don't listen to gossip." Lauren came in to the breakroom. "You're fear mongering, Camille. Break time is over, go back to your posts."

Lucky for Mindy, the shift was quiet on her first night. Maria and she had time to catch up.

"How's your academic adventure going?"

"The funding for minority scholarship was cut off after a year so I had to work as a grad assistant to help pay the tuition."

"So, you work at Northeastern, too?"

"It's only 10-hour a week. I like it, my boss is very nice. I learned a lot from her."

"You're really grinding it."

"It's okay, this Summer would be the final semester taking my last business class. Hopefully without a hitch, I would be graduating this September."

"Wow. I'm so proud of you, two masters. How did you do it? Working two jobs, studying and going through divorce."

"It's hard but I just don't think of how hard it is. Being busy, I ain't got no time for the pain, as the song goes. I bury them under heavy books."

"I always knew you have that quiet confidence in you to endure no matter what."

"Thanks Mindy. My teacher on this class, he's a visiting professor from Harvard. He laughed when, you know, on the first day he asked everyone to introduce themselves, I just blurted out, "Hi my name is Maria, I'm a part time nurse, part time student but a full-time mother."

"Haha, you've always been quick-witted. That's one thing I like about you."

"Aww, Mindy you're truly my friend."

Their conversation was interrupted when Mindy's admission came in. He's a 56 years old man from Chelsea working as a driver in the MBTA train. He seemed stable with minor symptoms. Maria helped her settle him down in the room, after which they just waited for the shift to end.

"That wasn't a bad first night." She commented as they walked out of the hospital together."

"No. Actually one for the books, as long as I can remember since I started there."

"By the way, they scheduled a picket this weekend. Will you join? I'll come if you are."

"Maybe. Not sure 100%. I don't have a placard.

"That's okay. Just being there to show support is enough. You can wear my T-shirt that says- 'I work in this shit-hole.'"

"Haha. Okay, I'll see you there."

Sunday afternoon, Maria and Mindy spent the time with the picketers. The street in front the hospital was clogged with hundreds of nurses milling around. They converged to the sides of the road to let vehicles drive through, honking their horns in response to the placard, 'Honk if you support the nurses.'

One sign says- 'Nurses dig the trenches in the battlefield of sick-care. We don't ask for the gold but just what's fair.'

Another says, 'You can't break our solidarity, we're ready to go on strike.'

While one placard spells out, 'She gets huge bonus, we get pizza?'

One says, 'No contract, no nurses to work the covid field.'

They were just walking up and down the streets in quiet protest when there was a small explosion on the far end of the road. Everybody scattered looking for safe place to hide. Luckily there was no one hurt. It wasn't meant to harm but just to scare nurses out of their wits.

"What a way to dissuade nurses from striking." Mindy exclaimed.

"Yeah, they are playing hard ball." Carol commented.

"Do they really think the scare tactics would change our minds?" Camille added.

The picketing ended prematurely and they parted ways but reminded each other to show up for the meeting and to vote yes. That night, instead of working on her class project, Maria wrote a letter to the VP of Nursing.

Dear madam,

As a nurse yourself, you know the risks that we face working day in and day out taking care of patients with diverse medical problems. But you're far removed from the bedside, the only risk you're exposed to is a paper cut.

Meanwhile, we deal with difficult patients, challenging work situations and psycho relatives that shows up armed to kill the staff. The nursing terrain is inhospitable, fraught with challenges laid out in a petri dish laced with covid-19 and other viral threats that spawn angst and anxiety every time we work the shifts.

You cannot pay us enough for the fear we faced every time we're stuck with a needle, when we enter a covid room praying we don't get sick, or when we get assaulted by a crazy patient. Maybe we should start asking for FEAR differential.

How much would the hospital pay for the fear that nurses experience in the work place? We're not asking to be compensated for the trepidation that comes with the job but only what's fair and equitable.

Respectfully,

Maria

She emailed it right away, hoping the Nursing VP would read it before nurses decide to strike. Whether it has an impact on her or not, at least she expressed what's in her mind.

Monday came, and Maria handed her ballot. She worked the night shift so she didn't stay for the whole meeting.

"Are you going now?" asked Carol.

"Yeah, I have to get some sleep before my class this evening."

"Okay, be careful driving home." Mindy said. "I'm staying till the end."

Maria walked to the garage, a little groggy from lack of sleep, but she noticed a guy in black hoodie following her. She stopped to look back and he stopped five yards behind her, pretending to look around. She walked faster, and entered the garage to find her car. The guy paused at the entrance then entered a red mustang convertible illegally parked on the side of the street. As she drove out, the red mustang followed her. She turned left on Brookline Avenue, and he did, too.

"Don't be paranoid." She told herself. Maybe he's just going the same way she does. But she remembered Camille telling them about a mysterious guy in black hoodie following and harassing nurses. Instead of turning left on Route 9 at the end of Brookline Avenue, which she usually takes to get to Jamaica way, she turned right to the opposite direction. She stepped on her gas pedal trying to lose him but he accelerated to catch up. He's now a few yards behind her and menacingly getting much closer for her comfort. Now she's close to panic mode.

"No harm can come to me. Where I Am, God is. Where God is, I Am. I am safe, I am protected." She repeated the mantra over and over again as she drove west on route 9 then exited taking High Street to get to Paul Pender Rotary on the Northern side of Jamaica Pond. She thought she lost the guy as he's no longer visible in her rearview mirror. She relaxed her knuckles and released her hands from its tight grasp on the steering wheel.

She took a big sigh of relief as she turned left on Chestnut Street. But as she approached the rotary, she saw the red car waiting right outside the circle where Pond Avenue ends to meet up with Chestnut Street. He must have taken Pond Avenue which is parallel to High Street and both end up to merge with the rotary traffic.

Now she's really scared. Without yielding to cars entering Paul Pender Rotary, she swerved in and drove faster to get to Perkins Street on the north shore of the tiny lake then turned left on Francis Parkman Drive curving around the western side of Jamaica Pond. As she was about to enter Arborway, the red car came up to her. He was on the other side of the pond. From Perkins Street he took Jamaica way, the road that runs along the eastern side of the pond, which also converge with Arborway. They both semi-circled the waterhole in the opposite sides; she drove the road on the west side while he was on the east, both streets leading to the tree-lined lanes of the Arborway. Boston streets make no sense. They intertwine and loop around without rhyme or reason and Maria looping around the senseless roads, she's grappling at the reason why this guy is following her.

Pedal to the metal, she drove top speed way above the speed limit. Now she's sure he's onto her. And he knew how she's going to get home.

"Why is she being targeted?" She asked herself. Was it because of the letter she wrote to the VP of nursing?

The Arborway lead to another rotary by the Arnold arboretum. She took Centre Street, the first exit out of the circle, instead of following Arborway all the way towards Forrest hills station, which was her usual route to get home. The guy in the red car was coming close behind her. She mumbled to herself, "Fear has no power over me. It dissolves in the light within."

She passed the Faulkner Hospital on the right side of Centre Street and a little farther is the Hebrew rehab center on the left side. Would she stop by one of these facilities? She wondered. Then she heard a voice.

"Take Centre Street all the way to the rotary by Holy Name Church."

Now, she had a plan. She headed towards the third rotary where a police station is located opposite the church on the other side of the circle. She stopped abruptly in front the inconspicuous building that looked like a regular residence. She entered the building, huffing and puffing.

"Hey, lady, what's going on. You look like a ghost." The clerk behind the front desk asked.

"I'm being followed by a guy in a red mustang." Maria was gasping for breath, and slumped herself in one of the chairs.

"I don't see any red mustang out there." He said walking to the front door peeking out the streets.

"I just came out from work. He followed me all the way here. He must have left."

"Can I get you some water or coffee?"

"I'm good thanks. Can I just sit here for some time before I drive home, make sure he's really gone."

"Take as much time as you need."

Maria was wired and tired from the chase but she managed to get home. She was glad she didn't have to go back to work tonight. She's reaching her saturation point where if she could quit her job tomorrow, she would. But she's in a bind; she has a mortgage to pay, a child to support, grad work to finish, and going through a divorce.

She slept for four hours then got ready for her 7 Pm class. Of all the different challenges she faced, whether it's emotional or physical, it's the intellectual challenge she doesn't mind. She thrived on it as it gave her freedom to explore the academic world and tap into the hidden resource within. It guided her to navigate through the comings and goings of her life.

All her grad projects, be it group presentation or individual papers required in every subject either in Nursing or business classes, she tackled them with uncertainty at first. But as she dug deep into her inner resources, she wings it with her mantra – 'Fake it till you make it.'

Tonight's power-point presentation was no different than the others. She didn't know how to go about the topic her group was given – Short term economic outlook of the US. It's a broad topic that required different factors that needed to be synthesized and organized as a coherent whole. But somehow, she's able to come up with a strategy to present it in a cohesive structure that's sensible and logical.

She entered the classroom late. The first group has already started their presentation.

"Maria, what kept you?" the leader of her group glared at her. "We were thinking you weren't gonna show up, and then we're screwed."

"Sorry, I can't find a parking space."

"We draw numbers to see who's presenting first. Thankfully we're the last one."

The professor divided the class into five groups with four members in each.

"I'm not quite ready with my slides. If you guys don't mind to go ahead with your part. I'll be the last."

There she goes again, cramming to the last minute. She told herself, nervously rearranging her notes.

"I shouldn't have drunk that much coffee beforehand." She chastised herself, her caffeinated hands shaking.

'You can do it, Maria. Just breathe! You live for this.' Says the soundless voice in her head. 'Remember, fake it till you make it.'

Her turn came, the last one in the last group to present. She stood behind the podium, nervous in front of the class with the visiting professor sitting on the left side of the last row. Maria thought he's probably comparing how Northeastern University students stack up with Harvard students. She dared not look where he was, just acknowledging her fellow students as she started her presentation. Her insides were trembling like a leaf as she opened with the title.

First slide: US Economic Outlook- What's Covid got to do with it? Everything!

Second slide: Factors influencing the US economy

1. GDP- gross domestic product, the primary measure for economic health.

2. Inflation – rate at which prices for consumers goods and services are rising.

3. Consumer spending – major drive to the economy based on household income and consumer confidence.

4. Unemployment rate – reflects the health of the labor market. High rates signal economic recession.

5. Fiscal policy – related to government spending and taxation.

6. Business Investments – reflect company's confidence in the future.

She's settling in her groove as she discussed each factor.

Third slide: Impact of the pandemic on the US economy.

1. GDP fell 3.5% - the 1st contraction since 2008 financial crisis, the biggest since 1946

2. Inflation rate – rise up to 6.2%, the biggest rise in 31 years.

3. Unemployment rate – sharp rise up to 20%, jobs down 14.6 million and those with jobs were dislocated from work place working remotely from home.

4. Consumer spending – with millions of people laid off, retail activity was grossly reduced.

5. Business/Investments – Collapse in the travel/ tourism industry and other small businesses. Financial markets - S&P and Dow Jones down significant points.

6. Fiscal Policy – Government spending increased with stimulus packages resulting to $3.1 trillion in public debt.

Now she's comfortable in her skin, as she went through each bullet point.

Fourth slide. Effects of Covid -19 across multiple sector;

1. Health sector – 25 million would lose their employer-provided health insurance with 7 million un-insured.

2. Increase in homelessness as eviction and foreclosures rise.

3. Food insecurity across the US – already prevalent pre-Covid with 17 million people lacking access to food supply. Up to 54 million citizens affected with disruption in shipping and supply chain.

4. Global Economic recession – with high inflation and unemployment rates, collapse of businesses and financial markets, recession was inevitable.

She took off paragliding above and beyond her own self-doubt and insecurity as she finished with the last slide:

The positive outcome. 'You never want a serious crisis to go to waste' - Winston Churchill.

1. Improved relationship – with enforced lockdowns, people learned to live together in harmonious way.

2. Ecological balance – Flora and fauna flourished with less people outside.

3. Air and water pollution reduced with less vehicles on the road.

4. More awareness on sanitation and hygiene.

5. Digital world was born with distance learning and tele-work became the norm.

Maria finished her presentation.

"With rising fatalities now over 103.4 million confirmed cases, and over 1.1 million confirmed deaths, the world is gripped in chaos and uncertainty. Humanity is about to be decimated and a portion of the population wiped out, but the major concern for some people is not food but toilet paper running out of grocery shelves. There's a rising TP insecurity as they are flying off the racks. What happened to just regular water to clean?"

The class laughed. Now that she's done, she looked at the professor, he was laughing, too.

Maria went back to her group, still shaky with adrenaline rush.

"Did you see the expression on the professor's face, Maria?" one member commented. "He was very impressed with you."

"No. I tried not to look at him."

The professor took back the podium to finish the class.

"Congratulations to all of you. You did a great job with your power point especially the last group."

The students started getting ready to leave.

"Before you go, I have an announcement about the finals. We only have two weeks for this summer semester and because you all did excellent work with the other requirements, I'm giving you an open book test. The questions are difficult in essay format so feel free to consult your textbook."

Maria went home satisfied but she wasn't prepared for the shock she was about to receive. Her mom died. In her deathbed she told her siblings to tell her not to fly home to the Philippines for the funeral. She knew Maria's finishing her graduate program. But how could she not see her one last time? She has to go even if that means she can't finish her last class. Unfinished class meant no grade, no grade no graduation for her, but she didn't care about any of it.

She called Mindy looking for emotional support. She's the only one in her life that gave her strength. She's the pillar that she leaned on when she felt unsteady and a stabilizing force when her world wobbled.

"I'm sorry to hear that, Maria."

"My mom doesn't want me to come home, but I have to."

"Definitely. Let me know what I can do for you."

"Thank you. I'll see you when I get back. Hopefully, the strike's over by then."

"I'm praying it won't happen. Anyways, I'll be here. And oh, by the way, when you get a chance, get me that dress I showed you from the magazine."

"Yes ma'am. Behave yourself while I'm away. Don't do anything. I wouldn't do."

She booked roundtrip tickets and told her nurse manager she'll be gone for some time. She gave her three weeks off from work. Now she has to tell her professor she can't finish his class.

Lucky for Maria he was a reasonable guy. He emailed her the test questions for her to work on where ever she might be. She packed her laptop and the textbook in her carry-on luggage and she headed for Logan airport. The Uber driver took her through the backroads hitting every red light before getting into the highway.

"Can you hurry up please, I'll be late for my flight."

"Can't do anything with the traffic miss. You know what they say, 'It takes an hour to drive from Boston to Boston.'"

Her flight out was at 7:45 pm, but with traffic congestion, she got delayed. After checking in she proceeded to the security line and was dismayed to see a sea of people in front of her. The overhead announcement came.

"Calling passengers for Delta flight 776. The gate will close in 15 minutes."

"Oh, shoot. There's no way I can make it to the gate with all these people." Exasperated, she slumped down behind an elderly lady trying to cram three hand carries into one.

"Miss, are you on this flight?" an attendant came up to her.

"Yeah, I'm afraid I can't make it to the gate in time." She replied standing up.

"Come with me." He replied, leading her to bypass all the passengers.

Like Moses, he parted the sea for her. He untied the black ropes separating the lines that looped around to get to the X-Ray machine. She didn't even have to go through it as she escorted her to the Delta gate.

"Hurry, hurry. You can make it."

And she did.

Maria lived for small miracles like this. More and more, as she's totally surrendered to a Higher Power, she sees the workings of a guiding Hand.

From Boston to Seattle, Seattle to Japan, as the plane crossed the Pacific, Maria got herself busy during the long flight answering the questions in her final exam. Thirty-three thousand feet above the ocean, she's in her last hurdle to complete her 84 hours total credits required for a dual-masters. Her mind was occupied for the most part of the 24-hour journey, poring over the textbook to find answers to the questions. On her last leg from Japan to Manila she couldn't concentrate as she's now consumed with grief.

Her younger sister picked her up from the airport and together with her three young kids, they drove 10 hours South of Manila to bury their mom. It was an emotional reunion seeing her sister and her children. It's been 14 years since she was last home. Raising a family, working, studying, life got in the way of connecting back to her roots. Life consumes life. She's here now but she wished it was for a happier occasion.

Her mom was laid out in a casket for 18 days. Her 82 years old body could no longer sustain her mortal life. She was embalmed to last that long as they waited for Maria and her two brothers working in merchant ships to come home. They were scheduled to arrive the next day, one's coming from Antarctica, one's from Africa, after which the funeral will take place. While waiting for them, Maria had the chance to sit with her mom in her last hours before they take her to the cemetery. She sat beside the casket, reminiscing her early childhood in a fishing village where her father used to operate a small boat, fishing the waters of South China sea. That was where her mom was assigned to teach for 20 years before she was transferred to a school in the town proper. Being the youngest at that time, she stayed with her parents in the village while her older siblings lived in their ancestral home in town.

The fishing village sits at the end of Bicol River, on the edge of nowhere but the barren waters of San Miguel Bay. Fishermen have to go farther into the deep reservoir of South China Sea to catch fish. The place was bleak and desolate except for few families living off the scant resources of the area ravaged constantly by typhoons. Their house, more solid and sturdier than most, situated a few meters off the shoreline would be the only one standing after a storm. The villagers would seek shelter with them, crammed up in the wooden house his father built. The rest, little nipa huts, swept away into the sea. She remembered as a child, seeing an elderly man with his dog, a rooster, and a little pig sitting on the thatched roof of a submerged shack slowly being pulled by the currents through the mouth of the river into the bay. He seemed calm, so too, were the animals with him, as if resigned to their impending doom.

The place may be dismal and harsh but for Maria, it was an idyllic setting for her formative years. Her childish affinity to the natural world fed her wild imagination. She'd make up stories in her mind and imagined herself building a bridge to cross the river into the next town, where her older brother would fetch gallons of drinking water. She never knew scarcity despite the lack of running water and electricity. The night was lit by the stars, bright against the black sky and all she saw in the dark were the flickering lights from the kerosene lamps glowing through small bamboo-framed windows of small shanties. Her father in his night trawling, going out at dusk in a small motorized boat, would come home early morning with a net-full of fresh fish still alive jumping up and down to get back to the water. He was versed with the many constellations, using the location of the stars in the night sky to guide him through the dark waters. He taught her how to spot the Orion belt, the Big Dipper, and the Pleiades. Although he was taken too soon from her, she still remembered the love, the joy as he carried her on his back, swimming farther from the shore to teach her how to swim. He was tough with his discipline but he was loving.

They were poor but they were supplied with bare necessities better than the others. They made do with what they have and she found comfort in the flowing river. She could stay in the water the entire day, if her parents would let her. She remembered making dolls molded out of the clay, dug out from the shoreline. She just had to be careful there's no brown turd mixed in with the grey mud. As a child she never knew there was a big world beyond the fishing village.

"I'm so sorry mom, I should have come home when you were still alive. Thank you for all the sacrifices you have made for me." Tears tainted with regrets and guilt could not be stopped.

She owed her life to her mom, not only for birthing her but saving her when they almost drowned in a boating accident. She was drifting off to sleep on the chair, lulled by the hum of the electric fan and the smell of the flowers in the room, when she felt her mom's hands lovingly held her left arm comforting her. Her touch triggered a vivid recollection of the incident. She was about 5 years old when the small boat they were in, carrying several blocks of ice turned sideways and capsized the boat in the middle of the deep river. The guy at the back operating the boat, didn't know how to swim and saved himself by climbing the top of the upturned canoe. Her mom, barely afloat in the water, grabbed the side of the boat with her left hand, clutching her water-filled handbag with her right. And as Maria was about to be swept away by the strong currents, she let go of her bag and grabbed her child with her free hand. She wouldn't let her daughter be taken away from her. She was hanging on to dear life- hers and her daughters- for some time before rescuers came. She could have died there and then but she didn't.

"Can I get you some coffee or food, maria?" Her older sister came up to her.

"No, thanks. I'm good."

"You've been sitting there for a long time. Go upstairs and take a nap. More people are coming to see her."

"I'm fine here for now." She couldn't be torn away from her mom.

"What time is the mass tomorrow?" She asked still dazed from the dream. "What's their ETA?"

"They're both in Manila now. They will be here early tomorrow. Mass was scheduled for 10 am."

She didn't sleep overnight. She was anxious to see her brothers which she hasn't seen for years. She owed it to both of them and grateful for their financial support during her college years. They sent money to her mom to pay for her tuition when most parents would sell their cows and farms to finance their kid's nursing education. Her second elder brother sacrificed going to college. After finishing high school, he joined the merchant marines with their oldest brother to support the family. They were like the older branches of a bush trimmed to allow for new growth to flourish. She was glad to see them again after a long time. This will be a bittersweet reunion, she told herself.

They arrived together at the crack of dawn, both travel bogged and grief-laden. Without sleep they all prepared for the longest journey they'll ever take, a mile and a half trek from their ancestral home to the cemetery where their beloved mother will be laid to rest.

There was already a long line of people following the procession when they started from her mom's house. But as they moved farther along from one barangay to another, more people were joining in to walk with them in the sweltering heat. There was a river of black umbrellas opened to shelter the mourning throng of townsfolks flowing through the streets. Maria was touched by how the whole town came to pay respect. She didn't know how big was her mom's impact on people's lives.

For their family, she was a beacon of light and hope. She was their beautiful princess; soft and gentle, yet strong enough to endure the hardships of raising nine children and working full time. She had an air of dignity about her as if she wasn't from this world. She didn't come here for a comfortable life. She came to transcend it and be okay in the discomfort. Her enduring legacy she left for them was embodying the most important lessons of all - integrity, humility and good will, and most of all to aspire for something better than the circumstance they were born in. Out of the goodness of her heart, she shared herself in quiet service to the people around her and serving the community at large. She was scattering her 'inner bread'. That was her dharma for which she didn't expect material gains.

The hearse advancing slowly in front of the family was playing her mom's favorite song- 'The Impossible dream.' It dug up an ache so deep in her heart, it took a herculean strength to control her tears. She remembered the lyrics as she used to sing it to her before sleep. "To dream the impossible dream, to fight the unbeatable foe. To bear the unbearable sorrow, to run where the brave dare not go. To right the un-rightable wrong, to love pure and chaste from afar. To try when your arms are to weary, to reach the unreachable star. This is my quest, to follow that star, no matter how hopeless, no matter how far. And I know if I'll only be true to this glorious quest, that my heart will lay peaceful and calm when I laid to my rest."

What was her impossible dream? Maria never knew. Maybe it was for her children to reach for the stars she never had the chance to in this lifetime. All she did was sacrificed her life to pave the way for them. She asked her once, which she regretted for years.

"Mom, if you're so smart graduating valedictorian in high school, how come you didn't use those smarts to make more money?"

She looked her in the eye lovingly and said, "Maria, money buys you comfort but it doesn't buy you character."

Maria followed her impossible dream and reached for her North star. She pursued a life away from her roots, traveled distant lands and while away, she has loved and lost and suffered the 'slings and arrows of outrageous fortune.' Now she's come full circle, returned home to find home isn't home anymore; not when her mom's gone. She realized time isn't linear. You don't go back to where you started and expect to find the same place. Rather, time is a spiral that loops around and returns at the place you started but at a different point in the swirl of time and space.

The heat in Philippines in early August was unforgiving. She wondered how she managed to walk the distance with sweat and tears mingling. Going back to the house, they took the local transport- a tricycle with a rickety side car that holds three people ideally, but cram more passengers on the back and side to accommodate ten. Living in the US with all the comfort and convenience, she'd forgotten the discomfort of the daily struggle to move along towards her goal. But that's how she learned patience and perseverance.

Maria and her sister drove back to manila while his two brothers stayed behind with the rest of the family. After two weeks without internet, she's able to get into her e-mails from Boston. She learned the hospital and the MNA settled the contract and nurses didn't have to strike. She was glad to hear the good news. There was an e-mail from Camille and Carol but none from Mindy. She's probably just busy with her kids, she thought. They usually spend time in Martha's Vineyard during Summer.

There were several urgent messages from Northeastern University. Her academic advisor asked:

"Maria, where are you? We've been calling your house phone and you're not answering. I've sent you several e-mails already. We haven't heard from you and we're a little worried. Call ASAP. We have to talk about your graduation."

She replied:

"I'm sorry I didn't tell you I was flying to the Philippines for my mom's funeral. I left in a hurry."

The college coordinator was asking:

"Maria, did you take your finals for Mr. Foster's class? He gave you an incomplete grade. You won't be able to join the September graduation on the 5th unless we receive your final grade."

"Yes, I did take the exam. I e-mailed it to him from the Philippines before the semester ended. He even gave me an A+."

"I'm glad to hear from you. He has to submit the official grade to his department and forward it to us. He's on vacation now somewhere, but don't worry, we'll hunt him down."

"Thank you so much! I'm flying back to Boston August 30. I hope I can still join the ceremony in September."

There was a string of e-mails going back and forth between Maria and the coordinator. Despite the 12-hour time difference, they were able to connect and work things out. Finally, she was in Japan waiting for her connecting flight to Seattle when she received the good news via e-mail.

"Maria, your professor submitted your final grade and you're all set for graduation."

That lifted her spirits up. After what she's been through, the Universe sends a rainbow to her storm. But the Universe was not done testing her mettle, yet.

The day after she arrived, she went to the city courthouse to finalize the divorce.

"I'm sorry to hear about your mom." Her husband soon to be ex offered his condolences.

"Thank you."

"You must be tired after a long flight."

"I'm okay, I slept most of the way."

"You must be glad this is finally over."

She just looked at him with tired eyes, jet-lagged from the long flight. It was a civil conversation between two people that got estranged by dysfunctional behavior and incompatibilities.

That night she came back to work, excited to see Mindy. She got her a Filipiniana dress. She's been asking Maria for it.

"Hey, Laura, Is Mindy on tonight?"She gave her a sad look. "Maria, brace yourself. She's gone."

"What do you mean she's gone? Gone where?" her knees starting to shake.

"She died a week ago. She got Covid while they were intubating her patient in room 301."

"Oh, God, Nooo!!!" Her world collapsed for the second time.

She was gone for three weeks to bury her mom, and came back to find her dear friend buried. This year has been the most horrible time in her life. Deaths and divorce in the midst of Covid pretty much summed up her annus horribilis.

Chapter Eleven

FROM FEAR TO FREEDOM

The days following her trip from the Philippines, she couldn't get herself to do anything. She was bogged down with mixed emotions - anger, sadness, fatigue. How much grief and sorrow can one take in one sitting? She asked God, the Universe, or whoever is in Charge. She's questioning her faith now. Is there really a Higher Power? If so, why does she feel abandoned. She's so overwhelmed and if not for her daughter she would have folded in the weight of her burden. She's desperately seeking for strength and demanding guidance from her invisible friend but she, too, seemed nowhere. She cannot hear her, not when she's outraged by everything that has happened in her life. All she heard was the howling of her wrath towards a vengeful god.

She remembered her guide saying, "You passed one test but there will be more."

Right now, she's spinning in a whirlwind of tests that's taking her into a dark tunnel. Is this what's life about? A passage through trials, one after another, navigating through a dark alley, then one day you wake up dead? What's the point of all these? She's got more questions than she can find answers to. And as she went through her dark night of the soul, her soul got darker.

She has suffered betrayal, disappointments, losses and now three deaths; two real ones and the third was the death of a relationship that has burnt its fire left unfed by a higher love. She felt like dying herself. She's drowning in a quick sand, pulling her down into the depths of desperation. Maria slept for two days, didn't care about the graduation coming up in two days. She was in a liminal space. She's here in Boston at the same time she's there in the fishing village in the Philippines being swept by the currents like the old man in the river. There was no resistance, just total surrender to where ever the stream would take her.

When she awakened, she's more settled into a peaceful state that allowed her to hear her guide.

"Maria, God walks with you even in your darkest hour. You don't feel it because you lowered your frequency with negative energies of grief, anger, despair. These are barriers to the Light that is ever present everywhere; omnipresent, omniscient, omnipotent. God and Light are one and the same. God is all there is. Light is all there is, and you are not separated from Him because Light is what you are, a spark of the Divine. You cannot hear me because you're veiled in shadows. You have to unveil yourself. Release anything not aligned with your essence which is pure light. What separates you from It, are the lower frequencies of negative emotions."

The graduation day came and went. It was the culmination of her hard work but the ceremony meant nothing to her now. She went through the motion and her mind and heart were not in it. She should be celebrating her accomplishment, but it felt empty. Flying back to Boston, she was looking forward to sharing the joy and excitement with her dear friend, Mindy. But she, too, was taken away. She wondered why she even bothered. Why did she pursue dual masters and for what? She did it, not for anybody but for herself, to stretch her capacity. It wasn't for anything but for the challenge of it.

It's like taking on the adversities of crossing the ocean, not for the destination, but for the experience of the waves and the winds against the sails; for the sense of freedom to explore what lies beyond; for the excitement of the adventure of being held in the vast ocean, floating in the uncertainty of the voyage, yet calm enough to face the gusty winds and to roll in with the swelling of the waves. And amidst the difficulties, be given the courage to go on.

For what transpired through the past year- the losses from the death of loved ones, the dissolution of her marriage- she needed more than courage to move on. She needed the strength to carry the weight of emptiness. She wondered what Tom, her gentle philosopher, would say to her. Not the usual cliché, "It's not what happened in life that matters but how you respond to it." He knew she's tired of hearing it.

What would his answer be to her question, "Is there a purpose to human suffering, is there meaning to it?"

Maria can hear him say, "life has no inherent meaning except for what we give it."

Maria wished she could see him as he whispered, "Take life as it comes and flow with the currents where ever it takes you. Walk the path of the pilgrim in whatever terrain appears in front of you."

She was getting ready for work when her academic advisor called.

"Hello Maria, you forgot to pick up your award. It's in my office."

"Oh? I didn't know about it."

"You didn't come to the after-ceremony dinner, so come get it when you got the chance.?

"I'm going to work tonight. But I'll swing by after work. Thank you."

The shift was quiet in the covid battle field. The unit felt like a tomb, eerily still, but on a micro level, it's swarming with unseen infectious critters.

"Hey Maria, you have an admission in room 302. Are you okay with it?" Carol, who's in charge now that Mindy was gone, informed her.

"Yeah, I'm good." She said with flat, bland response; no fear, no fuss.

She didn't care anymore about anything. Her spirit no longer engaged in the job. She's done.

After her shift, she stopped by Northeastern University to pick up her plaque.

"I'm so proud of you Maria. You did it! This award say's everything about your hard work." Her advisor beaming at her.

"Thank you so much for your help and guidance. It's greatly appreciated."

She drove home and went to sleep, didn't even look at the plaque that says: Northeastern University Graduate School of Nursing Presents this award of Excellence in Clinical Practice to Maria Valdez.

She slept through most of the day and she was still in bed when her daughter came in.

"Mom, it's 5 pm, aren't you going to work?"

"No, honey. I'm not working tonight."

"I unwrapped the thing you left in the living room table. Congratulations mama!"

"Thank you. Go get ready, tonight we're dining out in the most expensive restaurant in Bean town." And she hugged her so tight, hanging on to what's left in her life.

So, under the early Autumn skies, with the not-so-crisp air of mid-September, mother and daughter walked the cobbled-stone streets to the restaurant she always wanted to dine in but was afraid to be outcasted by the new Brahmin of Boston. Food was good, the ambiance was great overlooking the harbor. There was an air of opulence reminiscent of the old Brahmin culture, but gone was the snotty-ness of old elitism. The city has evolved into a hybrid of cultures from European and Asian immigrants with a mix of conservatism and liberalism. Maria, though, was neither conservative nor liberal. She walked the middle road, not subscribing to any ideology except for freedom.

The early settlers- the Puritans- came seeking freedom from religious persecution. Today's modern-day settlers came for economic opportunities, chasing the American dream. Some were lost in the dream, working two to three jobs to maintain big houses, expensive cars, and lavish lifestyle. But Maria was content with simple living. When most were obsessed with material wealth, she was chasing the uncommon fortune; the ability to reflect on one's misfortunes as they piled up in the spinning of time; pondering on why things happened and how it came to unfold in the fabric of her existence. But the why of things not as important as to how to transcend them.

Maria reflected on how far she had come. After all the hard times she went through, she's glad she still has her daughter to be grateful for and to celebrate life with. She realized it's the small victories and little triumphs in between the heartbreaks and grief that we appreciate life in its wholeness.

Her journey back to her ancestral roots, looking through the windows of her past, reliving the memories of childhood was cathartic. Her origins have influenced who she had become but doesn't identify who she is now and doesn't determine where she's going.

She's grateful destiny has brought her here of all places. She could have trekked the sand dunes of the middle east, breathing the dust of arid living; Or, she could have been in Europe, threading into the rich tapestry of European culture; Or worst, remained in the fishing village peddling the scarce bounty from the sea. But Providence swept her into the heart of Boston, the birthplace of freedom, from where the United States have spawned the rest of its territories. She explored New York city and Florida for alternate working posts and lived in Texas for a short while, but she kept coming back to Boston, her first love. With innate intellectual curiosity, she resonated with the cerebrally enhanced culture of the city. Dubbed the Athens of America, Maria enjoyed the ambiance of academic atmosphere surrounding the many Ivy-league schools in the area. She reveled in the historic charm and the fusion of the old and the new, the numerous museums and art galleries and mostly, the close proximity to the ocean.

Working at one of the leading hospitals in the city, Maria was grateful for the opportunity to expand her training as well as the adequate compensation to live in financial security. She plowed through the hard work because it paid the mortgage and kept her gainfully employed while thousands of people were losing their jobs during the pandemic and through bouts of economic recessions. But the seeds of discomfort sprinkled through the years has cracked, giving her a new perspective. When the work that once gave her meaning became just the job to put food on the table, it conflicted with her values. But if she quits her job, how would she and her daughter sustain their daily needs? When doubts crept in, she hears a comforting voice, "Be brave my child. You do not walk alone."

Through the years, she has matured emotionally and spiritually as she faced the many challenges. All the pain, bitterness, grief, heartbreaks composted year after year, now filtered through a new light of understanding. And from out of the muck of misery comes a new life, empowered to endure not just to survive but to thrive. Like the butterfly flapping its tender wings against the cocoon and in the struggle gained strength to fly out into the open, she evolved through pain and difficulties. Fear and strife were the catalyst to her growth. Now she's emerging from the chrysalis to realize fear kept her tightly in the cocoon. But she has outgrown it and ready to fly out to freedom!

That night she made one decisive action. She wrote a letter to her nurse manager giving her two-week notice. The death of her friend was not 'the straw that broke the camel's back' but the steel arrow that pierced her heart. It cracked open, wide enough to let in the light of deeper understanding. She has awakened to her own truth, that she no longer fit in the framework of conventional health care entrenched in the subterfuge of big pharma. Their drugs aimed not to cure but create more side effects that kept patients needing more drugs for the side effects. It's a profit driven business racking up a thousand percent gains from the production of their chemicals.

She's no longer resonating with the principles of traditional medical care which is fragmentary at best; dissecting the body like an experimental frog, separating it into different systems and organs instead of treating it as a whole. Medical practice is broken down into different specialties that at times lack congruence with each other's approach on how to manage a patient.

Maria thinks there's a better way to heal; less corrosive, more holistic and less damaging to the wallet. She's leaning towards emerging modalities in energy medicine that address the body-mind connection. Alternative modes of healing could be used to complement the traditional system but unfortunately, it's not accepted by hospitals that view it as woowoo. Some doctors are embracing this approach now but their numbers still not enough to change the tides towards wholistic health care. Furthermore, there has to be a shift in people's consciousness to embrace this method. Healing is a personal journey and whatever people resonate with, is their medicine.

Someone said, "Medical Science is a dying dinosaur." The evolutionary changes may not be too apparent for now, but Maria believed the future of healing arts lies in frequency and energy, of sound and light therapy. There are futuristic technologies like the Med-beds that have been dangled out to people who have lost faith in the current system of care, but seems elusive and too far out. But as more and more people embrace the alternative ways and reach a critical mass, the faster change could come to shift to wholistic health care.

The old system of chemical burn is not the ideal way to heal. But the collective consciousness may not be ready for the unconventional ways of healing. It has to evolve to a higher level and people have to align with it. Maria's inclined to join the 'lone ranger' club following the wisdom of trailblazers like Joe Dispenza, Bruce Lipton, Gregg Baden, who have found a way to help people heal independent of the conventional route.

She believed the body has an innate intelligence to heal itself given the right diet, exercise and balancing the lifeforce that flows through the intricate network of energy system within the body. According to Chinese Medicine, the body gets sick when there's an imbalance in the system. Any method that brings balance and coherence to mind and heart allows for health and well-being. There are over 37 trillion cells in the human body with a pulsating light and when these lights are activated, you become a powerhouse charged with the ability to bring homeostasis necessary for healing.

Just as the saying goes, 'you can't fight city hall', she realized she can't fight the system. The only thing she could do was walk away, as she found courage to break apart from what sustained her financially. Maria told herself, what good is financial security when your values are no longer aligned with it. She realized her relationship with work has become toxic, compromising her self-respect. Her insides were screaming for deliverance; plagued with bad headaches after a shift, feeling nauseous at work without apparent reason. Oftentimes she'd cry dreading the drive to the hospital and to make her feel better pretended each night shift would be her last. On the way to the unit, walking from the garage, she would sing – When tears are in your eyes, it's time to say goodbye.

And that's what she did. One fine Autumn morning, she broke the golden handcuffs that tied her to a cash cow. A big orange orb rising from the east greeted her as she walked out of the institution. The light of freedom shone exceptionally bright from the morning sun. She came out of the building, emerging from fear to freedom with a higher level of confidence despite the lack of certainty of what lies ahead. She realized that the triumph of all triumphs is the ability to transcend fear. Forged in the fires of challenging experiences, faith was her sword that cut through her fears and uncertainties. Now she understood what her guide once told her.

"I'll see you on the other side of fear."

She skipped to the garage like a child feeling light; free to walk the earth, unencumbered by the crippling angst of human existence for she knows she's supported, protected, provided for and loved beyond measure.

THE END

Sources:

NIH National Library of medicine

PMC -Pub Med Central

Journal Family Medicine and Primary Care

Biomed Central

New England Journal of Medicine

Healthline.com

www.ingramcontent.com/pod-product-compliance
Lightning Source LLC
LaVergne TN
LVHW050915210926
848482LV00012B/454
* 9 7 9 8 2 9 5 4 8 9 9 4 5 *